Clinician's Manual on
Intra-abdominal Infections

Clinician's Manual on Intra-abdominal Infections

Dr Thomas L Husted
University of Cincinnati College of Medicine
Cincinnati, Ohio,
USA

Prof. Dr. Hannes Wacha
Hospital zum heiligen Geist
Academic Hospital of the University of Frankfurt
Frankfurt,
Germany

Professor Joseph S Solomkin
University of Cincinnati College of Medicine,
Cincinnati, Ohio,
USA

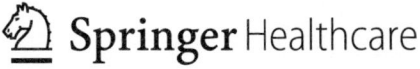

Published by Springer Healthcare Ltd, 236 Gray's Inn Road, London, WC1X 8HL, UK

www.springerhealthcare.com

©2010 Springer Healthcare, a part of Springer Science+Business Media

British Library Cataloguing-in-Publication Data.

A catalogue record for this book is available from the British Library.

ISBN 978-1-85873-188-9

Although every effort has been made to ensure that drug doses and other information are presented accurately in this publication, the ultimate responsibility rests with the prescribing physician. Neither the publisher nor the authors can be held responsible for errors or for any consequences arising from the use of the information contained herein. Any product mentioned in this publication should be used in accordance with the prescribing information prepared by the manufacturers. No claims or endorsements are made for any drug or compound at present under clinical investigation.

Commissioning editor: Ian Stoneham
Project editor: Lisa Langley
Designers: Joe Harvey and Taymoor Fouladi
Production: Marina Maher

Contents

Author biographies		vii
Preface		ix
1	**Assessing and evaluating the patient**	**1**
	Medical history	1
	Physical examination	1
	Laboratory studies	4
	Imaging	4
	Resuscitation prior and during intervention	5
	Options for intervention	5
2	**General management issues**	**7**
	Source control	7
	Wound management	9
	Nutrition	10
	Management of underlying pathology	10
	Post-operative management	10
3	**Diagnosis and management of specific diseases**	**13**
	Peptic ulcer	13
	Acute cholecystitis	16
	Acute cholangitis	20
	Acute/complicated pancreatitis	22
	Acute appendicitis	26
	Ischemic colitis	30
	Diverticulitis	33
	Inflammatory bowel disease	37
	Clostridium difficile colitis	42
	Post-operative intra-abdominal processes	44
	Post-operative superficial wound infection	50
4	**Antimicrobial management**	**51**
	Introduction	51
	Empiric antibiotic treatment	57
	Therapeutic antimicrobial treatment	58
	Antibiotic treatment and outcome	63
	Special considerations	64
Appendix		**69**
Suggested reading		**77**

Author biographies

Thomas L Husted, MD is a Surgical Resident in Critical Care Medicine, and Clinical Lecturer, in the Department of Surgery, at the University of Cincinnati College of Medicine, Cincinnati, USA. He obtained his bachelor degree at the University of Michigan, and completed his medical training at Wayne State University School of Medicine, Michigan, USA. Following this, he undertook an internship in general surgery at the University of California, USA, before joining the US Navy. After completing his service, he began a surgical residency at the University of Cincinnati College of Medicine. He has also been a research fellow at The Laboratory of Trauma, Sepsis & Inflammation Research, and a fellow in surgical critical care at the University of Cincinnati College of Medicine. Dr Husted has authored and contributed to a number of books, and peer-reviewed journals. He is also a member of the American College of Surgeons, the Association for Academic Surgery, the Society of Critical Care Medicine, and the Society of American Gastrointestinal and Endoscopic Surgeons.

Hannes Wacha, MD is Professor of Surgery, and Clinical Lecturer in the Department of Surgery, at the Hospital zum heiligen Geist of the University of Frankfurt, Academic Hospital of the University of Frankfurt, Germany. He is also Head of the Department of General Surgery, which includes the Trauma and Orthopaedic Surgery Unit, at the Hospital zum heiligen Geist. He completed his medical training in 1968, and subsequently took up a number of clinical posts at several institutions, including the Institute of Pathology, Departments of Thoracic & Vascular Surgery, General Surgery, and Trauma, at Northwest Hospital, Frankfurt, Germany, and the Clinic of Internal Medicine at the Holy Spirit Hospital of Frankfurt. Following this, he took up a teaching post at the University of Frankfurt, which he currently holds. He subsequently became Professor of Surgery in the Department of Surgery at the Hospital zum heiligen Geist, a position he has held for over 20 years.

Professor Wacha holds numerous memberships to several surgical societies, including the German Surgical Society, the International Society of Surgery, the Paul–Ehrlich Foundation, the American Surgical Infection Society, and the Surgical Infection Society of Europe (SIS-E). He was appointed Chair of the National Representative Committee of SIS-E (1996), and President (2006–7). He was also Vice-President of the Paul–Ehrlich Foundation (1999). Professor Wacha has written extensively and has authored and contributed to a number of publications. His main research interest is surgical infectious disease.

Joseph S Solomkin, MD is Professor of Surgery and Director of Research in the Division of Trauma and Critical Care at the University of Cincinnati College of Medicine, Cincinnati, USA. After graduating from Harvard College, Massachusetts, USA, and completing medical school and an internship at The Albert Einstein College of Medicine - Bronx Municipal Hospital Center, New York, USA, he went into the US Army Medical Corps. After his service he completed a surgical residency at the University of Minnesota, Minneapolis, USA (1973), serving as Associate and Chief Resident from 1977–1979. Following work at Piper Memorial Hospital in Zaire, Professor Solomkin had a fellowship in surgical infectious diseases at the University of Minnesota. He has been Assistant and Associate Professor in the Department of Surgery at the University of Cincinnati College of Medicine (1981–1994).

Professor Solomkin has authored and contributed to a broad range of international publications. He is active in numerous professional organizations. His principal areas of interest are infectious diseases in surgical and intensive care.

Preface

Advances in medicine and medical technology have had a significant impact on the treatment of intra-abdominal infections, and have enabled less invasive procedures to be carried out. Nevertheless, surgical procedures are still recognized today, to be one of the most effective means to treat intra-abdominal infections. However, prior to 1876 this was far from current thinking; it was believed that the peritoneum was unassailable. This assumption was first contradicted by Wegener at the 1876 German Congress of Surgeons, and by the first surgical closure of a perforated ulcer and appendectomy carried out by Mikulicz–Radecki in 1885. The first surgical appendectomy was also thought to be carried out around this time. These simple procedures – appendectomy and suture – contributed significantly to a dramatic change in mortality and wound infection rates over the years. Mortality rates fell from 90% to 20–60% (depending on the cause of diffuse peritonitis), and in perforated cases of appendicitis, mortality fell from 35% to 0%. Nowadays, death from appendicitis is fortunately rare; in the authors' experience there have been no deaths in the past 20 years from diffuse peritonitis following appendicitis. In addition morbidity today, due to abscess and wound infection rates, has also fallen considerably (eg, from 50% to 1–3%).

So how then have surgical procedures in the treatment of intra-abdominal infections developed? The answer is largely through experience, simply by being carried out in daily surgical practice, and adopted without the application of any particular study design. One example is the use of primary intention in wound healing. Before the introduction of antibiotics wound healing by second intention was the preferred surgical procedure, and involved the healing of an open wound by laying new tissue over the wound, as opposed to primary intention where the edges of the surgical incision are closed together using stitches or surgical clips, until the skin is healed and the cut edges have merged.

Today, however, primary closure is done in almost every case. The past 20 years have seen a marked shift in surgical practice toward primary intention as more effective and modern antibiotics have become available. While this is standard practice today, it is speculated by some that wound healing by second intention is still being practiced in many parts of the world. Most importantly, while the choice of surgical procedure will depend on a number of factors, the best outcome is always achieved when, following a correct diagnosis, the patient is found to be in need of an operation, and this operation is subsequently performed in a timely manner using the most appropriate surgical procedures for the encountered pathology.

In daily practice, however, it is not always easy to determine the correct diagnosis; the indication for an operation is often based on a suspected or hypothetical diagnosis. In spite of this, the decision to intervene is usually the right one, although it is possible that one may encounter another pathology than originally anticipated (eg, in patients with acute abdominal infection, one may find a variety of causes for the infection).

While advances in surgery have reduced mortality and wound infection rates in the treatment of intra-abdominal infections, what has been the role of antibiotics? The introduction of antibiotics shortly after the clinical experiment to open up the abdomen was also significant. The use of antibiotics, together with surgery and intensive care measures, further reduced mortality and wound infection rates. For example, before the antibiotic era mortality was 5–35%. The introduction of antibiotics saw this rate decrease to less than 14% between 1944 and 1986, and saw wound infection rates decrease to 10–58% (using ampicillin, cephalosporin, gentamycin, tetracycline, and kanamycin), with a mortality rate for abscess formation after appendectomy of 5–20%. Today, the use of more effective combinations of broad-spectrum antibiotics active against anaerobes has resulted in even lower rates of infection (eg, 4–7% for abscess formation after appendectomy).

The basic principles of rapid diagnosis, timely physiologic support and definitive intervention for intra-abdominal infections, have remained unchanged over the past century, yet the specific management of these conditions has been transformed by developments in medical technology. Newer approaches in radiologic techniques, intensive care medicine (anesthesia) surgery and the development of new minor-traumatizing techniques, and antibiotic coverage have resulted in an ever-growing complexity of management. There is no doubt therefore that these different therapies combined are, and will continue to be, the keystone of reducing mortality and bacterial complications in intra-abdominal infections.

This manual is intended for residents and physicians occupied in non-surgical disciplines who may become involved in the care of surgical patients. Recently, several guidelines have been developed for the diagnosis and management of a number of conditions including suspected acute appendicitis, acute cholecystitis and diverticulitis. These infections are the bulk of community-acquired intra-abdominal infections encountered in practice. I believe that this book will help many physicians to quickly recognize and understand the pathogenesis of intra-abdominal infections better, which will not only improve patient care but also provide the reader with intellectual satisfaction. It is our hope that the simple format of this book, along with the illustrations, will form an essential and quick reference guide for all non-surgical residents and physicians.

Hannes Wacha, Frankfurt, 2010

Chapter 1

Assessing and evaluating the patient

Medical history

The ideal starting point for discussion is the patient who presents to hospital with severe abdominal pain and evidence of intra-abdominal inflammatory disease (*see* Figure 1.1). The characteristics of abdominal pain that are most revealing are the time of onset, the location and radiation of the pain, and any provocative or palliative factors. Associated symptoms that should also be elicited are different types of pain (eg, colic or constant), nausea or vomiting, fever, anorexia, diarrhea or bloody stools, and dysuria.

Significant medical history includes any previous abdominal operations or trauma, a known presence of cholelithiasis or diverticulosis, cardiovascular disease, diabetes mellitus, inflammatory bowel disease or HIV infection. Pertinent social history includes tobacco and alcohol use. Other important factors to consider when taking a medical history include current medications and known drug allergies, recent travel history, and a complete review of symptoms.

Physical examination

With repeated examination and observation over time, the patient's general appearance and behavior should also be noted – appearing ill, malnourished, lying still or unable to find comfort are all factors that should be considered. The back may reveal Grey–Turner's sign of necrotic pancreatitis or the costovertebral tenderness of pyelonephritis. A careful cardiopulmonary exam is necessary to exclude cardiac and respiratory causes of abdominal pain. The abdomen is classically examined in four stages:

- inspection;
- auscultation (eg, bowel sounds);
- no bowel movement for 24–36 hours; and
- percussion and palpation.

Recognition and management of intra-abdominal infections

Patient has suspected intra-abdominal infection

Obtain history, including previous surgical manipulation of abdomen
Perform physical examination, focusing on abdomen, pelvis and vagina, and rectum (inspection, auscultation, percussion, palpation)

Order blood tests as appropriate:
• General tests of systemic response to infection
• Specific tests to localize source or focus of infection
On occasion, a young patient with classic presentation of appendicitis may be taken to the OR without blood tests or imaging

Order diagnostic imaging as appropriate

Patient has 'certain' appendicitis	History and physical exam warrant exploration of abdomen for peritonitis, but confirmation (free air) is needed first; or index of suspicion for peritonitis is very low	Patient has upper abdominal pain, elevated bilirubin level or liver function test results, or history of biliary tract disease	All other patients
Resuscitate, give antibiotics, and take to the OR	Obtain plain, abdominal films, including upright chest film	Order upper abdominal US, treat specific infection as appropriate	Order abdominal and pelvic CT scans, treat specific infection as appropriate

Free peritoneal air is present	No free peritoneal air is present, and index of suspicion for peritonitis is low	No free peritoneal air is present, but index of suspicion for peritonitis is high
Resuscitate, give antibiotics, and take to the OR	Discharge from surgical care	Order abdominal and pelvic CT scans (see above right)

Figure 1.1 Recognition and management of intra-abdominal infections. CT, computed tomograpy; OR, operating room; US, ultrasound. Reproduced with permission from Sawyer et al. Recognition and management of intra-abdominal infection. In: ACS Surgery: principles and practice. Edited by DW Wilmore. New York: WebMD, 2004; 1–29.

The location and severity of pain is noted (Figure 1.2) and the abdomen is assessed for localized or generalized peritonitis (Figure 1.3). A rectal exam in all patients complaining of abdominal pain is important to determine the presence of pelvic pain and blood, slime, or mucus in the stool (eg, in the case of diverticulitis).

The main symptom of intra-abdominal infection is pain		
Where is the pain?	**Type of pain**	**Possible diagnosis**
Entire abdomen	Gradual onset, progressing in severity, persistent (<6 h)	Illness of great importance severity, usually requires surgery
Upper abdomen		
Upper abdomen (epigastric region)	Sudden in onset, sharp, burning, severe, with/without abdominal defense	Often correlates with perforation of viscus (peptic ulcer perforation)
Right upper quadrant	Original localization, upper right, shifting to the back (right shoulder)	Acute cholecystitis, choledochal stone obstruction (cholangitis)
Right to the left upper abdomen	Shifting to the left costal margin (like a belt, semicircular)	Acute pancreatitis
Lower abdomen		
Right or left abdomen	Shifting from the flank to groin and testicle, cramping intermittent, intervals	Urethral calculi
Right or left lower quadrant	Cramping intermittent type short interval (relieve by vomiting)	Small bowel obstruction
Right or left lower quandrant	Cramping intermittent type, later dull	Diverticulitis, perforated tubo-ovarian cyst (abscess)
Left lower quadrant	Cramping intermittent, later dull	Sigma diverticulitis, (abscess-perforation)
Right lower quadrant	Original localization navel shifting to the right and to the lower abdomen	Acute appendicitis
Lower abdomen, entire abdomen	Abdominal pain shifting to the back	Ruptured aneurysm of the aorta

Figure 1.2 The main symptom of intra-abdominal infection is pain. There are many different diagnoses which can cause acute abdominal pain. In a study of 10,320 patients, the majority of patients presenting with acute pain in the abdomen had an intra-abdominal infection. Data from Lankisch et al. [Certified medical education: the acute abdomen from a medical point of view]. Dtsch Arztebl 2006; 103: A2179–88 and de Dombal FT. Diagnosis of acute abdominal pain. New York: Churchill Livingstone 1991.

Types of peritonitis		
Type of peritonitis	Cause/source/spread (diffuse or localized)	Examples/ spread (diffuse or localized)
Primary (spontaneous bacterial peritonitis)	Diffuse bacterial infection without an intra-abdominal source of infection (extraperitoneal source)	Pneumococcal infection in immunosupressed patients. Predisposed are children under 10 years of age, patients with ascites, liver cirrhoses (prevalence 8–12%), lupus erythematosus, nephrotic syndrome
Secondary	Bacterial contamination from a known source, perforation of the gastrointestinal tract Most common infection in surgery	Perforated appendicitis, abscess formation or diffuse spread of the infection as in the case of diverticulitis, postoperative peritonitis (eg, anastomotic leakage), special infection due to foreign bodies like catheters (eg secondary peritonitis in peritoneal dialysis)
Tertiary (defined as ongoing intra-abdominal infection after adequate treatment)	Persistent or recurrent infection after primary or secondary peritonitis	Ongoing peritonitis with abscesses after eradication of the source of infection and antibiotic therapy, nosocomial infection is most common in the 'open abdomen', overgrowth with multiresistant organisms and *Candida* spp.

Figure 1.3 Types of peritonitis. Data from Mazuski and Solomkin. Surg Clin North Am 2009; 89:421–37 and Wacha et al. [Peritonitis and other intra-abdominal infections]. In: Die Infektiologie. Edited by Adam et al. Berlin: Springer, 2004; 333–52.

Laboratory studies

Laboratory tests are categorized into general and specific investigations. General tests include a complete blood count, metabolic panel, C-reactive protein (CRP), and procalcitonin test. Specific evaluations include liver function, pancreatic enzymes, urinalysis and serum lactate level tests. In patients who are severely ill, blood cultures and an arterial blood gas are also carried out.

Imaging

Non-specific imaging includes a chest X-ray to exclude pulmonary causes of abdominal pain, or free air under the diaphragm (detected in 60% of perforations), which would indicate viscous perforation. Abdominal X-rays are obtained to detect any bowel obstruction (eg, distended small bowel loops, gas-fluid levels, absence of gas in the colon), volvulus, or the pneumatosis of mesenteric ischemia.

Specific diagnostic imaging includes abdominal and pelvic ultrasonography or computed tomography (CT), with or without contrast agents. At present, CT is the most sensitive and specific imaging modality available. Abdominal ultrasonography is very sensitive in detecting even minimal fluid collections and is useful for detecting biliary disease and gynecologic disorders of the pelvis, while abdominal CT is able to assess for acute appendicitis, diverticulitis, complicated pancreatitis, bowel obstruction, mesenteric ischemia, and abdominal aortic aneurysm. Moreover, CT also allows non-operative (interventional) management to be used as the definitive therapy (eg, expectant treatment of simple perforated duodenal ulcer).

Upper and lower endoscopies also play a very important role in detecting peptic ulcer disease, and diverticulosis.

Resuscitation prior and during intervention

All patients with acute abdominal pain will benefit from initial bowel rest, intravenous hydration and pain control – all of which should be initiated during the diagnostic procedures. Initial laboratory results will guide the use of transfusions in resuscitation. Moreover, whilst empiric administration of antibiotic therapy is tempting, caution should be exercised unless the patient is in extremis.

Options for intervention

Depending on the final diagnosis, patients may be suitable for medical therapy, radiologic intervention, or immediate surgical intervention. Each patient and each diagnosis should receive careful consideration regarding the appropriate initial intervention. Occasionally, administration of systemic antibiotics is all that is necessary, as in the case of spontaneous peritonitis or ischemic colitis. Simple abscesses can be treated adequately with simple aspiration and antibiotics. Discrete fluid collections, however, may require a percutaneous indwelling drain to be placed under radiographic guidance. Operative management (either open or simple laparoscopic closure) is employed for the resection of damaged or inflamed and unsalvageable organs, diversion of enteric contents, or drainage of collections that are too thick or numerous for percutaneous drainage.

Chapter 2

General management issues

Source control

Patients with intra-abdominal infection require source control – debulking of the infectious inoculum to such a degree that antibiotic therapy and host defenses are able to clear the bacterial contamination and restore normal homeostasis. When defining source control it is important to differentiate between:

- control of the source of infection (eg, closure of a hole in the viscus);
- resection (eg, appendectomy, cholecystectomy, sigma resection);
- colon deviation to exclude the source of infection; and
- clearing the abdomen from visible fibrin and necrotic tissue.

Source control procedures can vary (eg, in Europe and the USA, between hospital departments); however, once the infection has spread over the entire body, they are of limited value. At present there is no generally accepted definition of source control; however, the definition provided by Marshall (2004) encapsulates the key issues in defining source control:

- drainage of abscess or infected fluid collection;
- debridement of necrotic infected tissue; and
- definitive measures to control sources of ongoing microbial contamination and restore anatomy and function.

Intra-abdominal sources of infection that require control are infected fluid collections, abscesses, and (sterile or infected) necrotic tissue. Two approaches are available for source control: open and percutaneous.

Open

Surgical control of infection involves laparotomy or laparoscopic exploration to detect and close, or eradicate the source of infection. Debridement of necrotic tissue, drainage of abscesses or infected fluid collections, and copious irrigation of the abdominal cavity, can also be done (*see* Figure 2.1). However, although debridement has long been considered necessary to facilitate healing, its benefit has not been proven; similarly, the benefits of vigorous irrigation remain unproven, and although it causes no harm, it may be unnecessary.

The open approach is seldomly selected in modern surgical practice given the advent of radiographically guided drainage of intra-abdominal sources of infection.

Percutaneous

Radiographically guided drainage of intra-abdominal sources of infection has effectively replaced surgical exploration for source control (*see* Figure 2.2). Either ultrasound- or CT-guided drainage can be performed through the abdominal wall or through natural orifices, such as the rectum or vagina.

Minimally invasive percutaneous drainage has significantly improved results over open surgical drainage; it has resulted in lower morbidity rates and shorter healing times. Any fluid obtained from percutaneous drainage should be collected and cultures performed to determine sterility or infection and to guide antibiotic therapy.

Necrotic debris being removed from a patient with infected pancreatitis

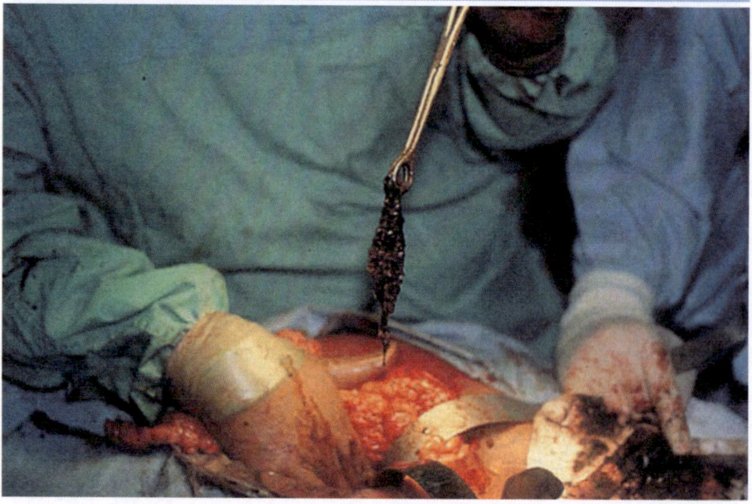

Figure 2.1 Necrotic debris being removed from a patient with infected pancreatitis. The main therapeutic approaches to pancreatic abscess are surgical debridement and drainage, percutaneous drainage, and antimicrobial therapy. From Finegold et al. Intra-abdominal infections and abscesses. In: Atlas of infectious diseases: intra-abdominal infections, hepatitis, and gastroenteritis. Edited by G Mandell, B Lorber. Philadelphia: Current Medicine LLC, 1997.

Left phrenic abscess being drained percutaneously

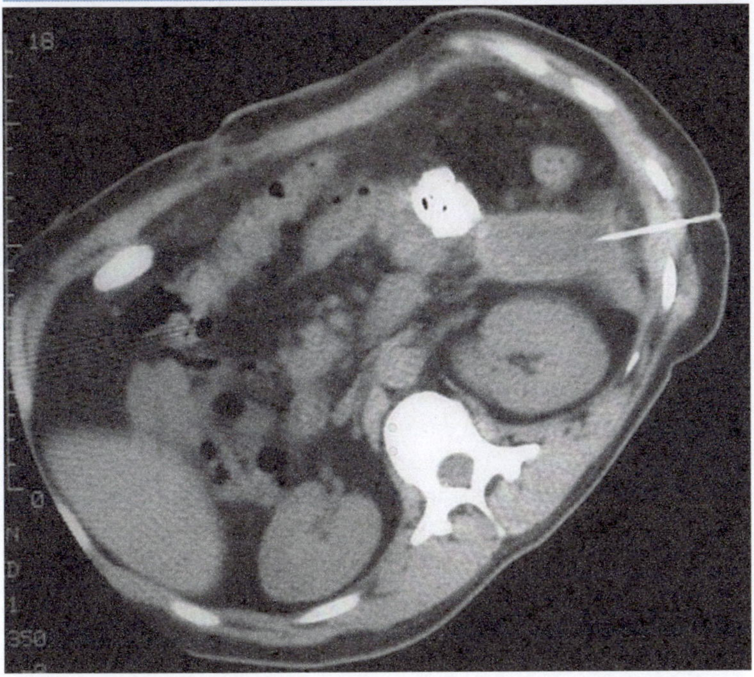

Figure 2.2 Left phrenic abscess being drained percutaneously. The needle can be seen in the abscess cavity on the right of this CT scan. Perinephric abscess is an uncommon complication of urinary tract infection and usually occurs secondary to obstruction or, occasionally, bacteremia. CT scan and, to a lesser extent, renal ultrasound have improved our capability of early diagnosis considerably. In addition to antimicrobial therapy, drainage is important. In most cases, patients do well with percutaneous drainage; if this fails, surgery is necessary. From Finegold et al. In: Atlas of infectious diseases: intra-abdominal infections, hepatitis, and gastroenteritis. Edited by B Lorber. Philadelphia: Current Medicine LLC, 2000.

Wound management

Traditional teaching mandates that abdominal incisions created to drain or address infected intra-abdominal processes are left open to heal by secondary intention. However, this is extremely rare in practice and it is seldom done in Europe, except in cases of diffuse peritonitis without source control, where it is necessary in up to 10% of cases. Once the peritoneum is copiously irrigated, the abdominal wall fascia is reapproximated and the skin edges are left open. Current practice makes use of open foam packing and closed suction devices. The use of vacuum-assisted closure devices has resulted in reduced morbidity by lessening the incidence of wound infections, gastrointestinal fistula and the need for reoperative closure. In addition, vacuum-assisted closure devices result in a significantly improved cosmetic outcome.

Nutrition

While nutritional concerns are valid in every patient, those presenting with infectious or inflammatory intra-abdominal processes usually suffer from some degree of ileus (intestinal obstruction). It is recommended that patients are kept at bowel rest, with the aim of restoring bowel movement and normalizing gut function, unless there is a substantial loss of the contents of the gastrointestinal tract or in cases of fistula. Most processes, however, require optimal nutrition in order to heal, which can present a problem as basic surgical premise supports using the gastrointestinal tract for nutrition if at all possible, either through normal dietary intake or via the use of nasoenteral feeding tubes (ie, enteral feeding). In those rare patients unable to tolerate enteral feeding or in which enteral feedings are contraindicated, then parenteral nutrition is an alternative choice. While the risks and benefits of parenteral nutrition are beyond the scope of this book, it should be acknowledged that in nearly all cases, enteral nutrition is preferred, better tolerated and more physiologic than parenteral nutrition, which can result in:

- mucosal atrophy;
- gut barrier dysfunction;
- reduction of the immunodefense system;
- translocation of organisms from the gut; and
- impairment of local bacterial defense mechanisms.

Management of underlying pathology

Regardless of the cause of intra-abdominal infection, the initial resuscitation and therapy are usually similar, and are based on intravenous fluid administration, bowel rest, and empiric antibiotic therapy. However, the specific pathologic disease process must be identified early and disease-specific therapy initiated. Disease-specific therapy may range from surgical resection in acute appendicitis and interval surgical intervention in acute cholecystitis, to non-operative medical therapy in ischemic colitis.

Post-operative management

Care of the post-operative patient following drainage of an intra-abdominal infection is very similar to general post-operative patient care. Specific concern is warranted in relation to improvement of infectious signs and symptoms. Expected events include resolution of fevers, normalization of leukocytosis, decrease in drain output, and improvement of any signs of sepsis. Antibiotic therapy should continue for a time after signs of improvement are recorded; however, this time should be as short as possible. Antibiotic treatment should be reconsidered after 3–5 days (counting the operation day as the first day), changed only when, according to the susceptibility tests, the outcome is poor, and stopped when bowel movement is achieved.

Any failure to improve after attempted source control for intra-abdominal infection should prompt an immediate search for inadequate drainage, recurrent infection or necrosis, a synchronous cause of infection or inflammation.

Chapter 3

Diagnosis and management of specific diseases

Peptic ulcer

Pathophysiology

The majority of mucosal ulcers are associated with *Helicobacter pylori* infection or ingestion of non-steroidal anti-inflammatory drugs (NSAIDs) (*see* Figure 3.1), although this has decreased in incidence since the advent of histamine H_2-receptor antagonists and proton pump inhibitors. Ulcers can lead to obstruction, hemorrhage, or perforation.

Medical history and physical examination

Patients with ulcer disease complain of dyspeptic symptoms (epigastric discomfort, nausea, belching, or bloating). Pain is the most common symptom (*see* Figure 3.2) and is usually relieved with eating, although a decrease in appetite may be reported. Examination may be unrevealing, although a positive stool guaiac test may suggest a bleeding upper gastrointestinal ulcer. Pain that is sudden and severe, accompanying abdominal rigidity, suggests perforation of a gastric or duodenal ulcer.

Laboratory studies

Ulcer disease may lead to anemia from chronic bleeding. Acute perforation of an ulcer may reveal leukocytosis. In cases of multiple ulcers or severe recurrent disease, a diagnosis of gastrinoma must be entertained. A gastrin level greater than 1000 mg/mL after cessation of therapy with H_2-receptor antagonists or proton pump inhibitors is suggestive of gastrinoma, requiring a diagnostic work-up for Zollinger–Ellison syndrome.

Diagnostic imaging

The simplest imaging to obtain is the upright chest X-ray (*see* Figure 3.3). In cases of ulcer perforation with free air in the abdomen causing abdominal pain, the chest X-ray will reveal air under the diaphragm in approximately 70% of patients. Contrast studies (in the absence of perforation) will demonstrate ulcers and are complementary to endoscopy for definitive diagnosis and obtaining biopsies.

Confirming the diagnosis

Ulcer disease is confirmed under direct visualization using endoscopy. Four-quadrant margin and central biopsies are obtained to assess for *H. pylori* and carcinoma.

Resuscitation

Patients with complicated ulcer disease may require intravenous hydration as well as transfusion, infusion of acid anti-secretory medications, and correction of any coagulopathy.

Interventional approaches

Non-operative

Uncomplicated ulcer disease can be treated non-operatively with cessation of NSAIDs, treatment of *H. pylori* infection if present, and therapy with a

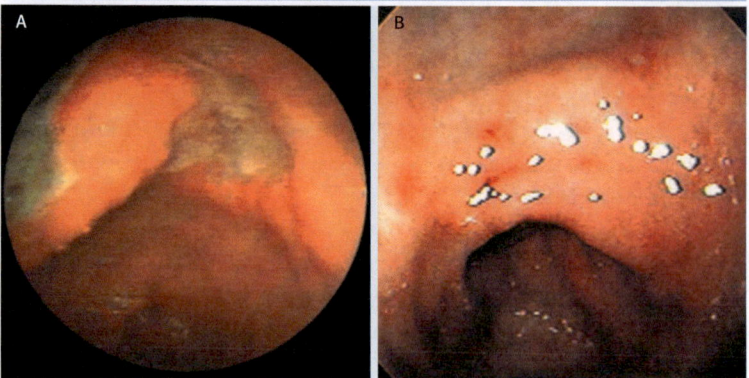

Ulcer disease associated with *Helicobacter pylori* infection and ingestion of NSAIDs

Figure 3.1 Ulcer disease associated with *Helicobacter pylori* infection and ingestion of NSAIDs. NSAID, Non-steroidal anti-inflammatory drugs. **A,** Irregularly shaped gastric ulcers at the angulus incisura. Biopsy showed well-differentiated gastric lymphoma. Biopsies of surrounding mucosa showed *Helicobacter pylori* infection. The lesions resolved with treatment of *H. pylori* infection. From Graham et al. Atlas of infectious diseases: intra-abdominal infections, hepatitis, and gastroenteritis. Edited by G Mandell, B Lorber. Philadelphia: Current Medicine LLC, 1997. **B,** Ulcer disease due to ingestion of NSAIDs. From Wilcox C. Gastroenterology and hepatology: stomach and duodenum. Edited by M Feldman, Philadelphia: Current Medicine LLC, 1996.

Clinical manifestation of ulcer disease

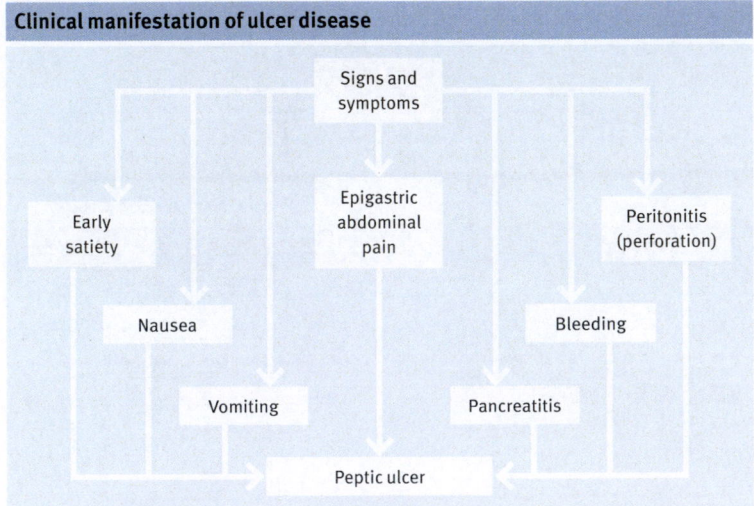

Figure 3.2 Clinical manifestation of ulcer disease. The most common finding on presentation of both gastric and duodenal ulcers is abdominal pain. The pain is usually localized to the epigastrium, although it may be located in the right upper quadrant (duodenal ulcer) or the left upper quadrant (gastric ulcer). Pain typically occurs between meals or at night in patients with duodenal ulcer but can be seen in gastric ulcer as well. Unusual presentations of ulcers include chest or back pain or pancreatitis. From Wilcox C. Gastroenterology and hepatology: stomach and duodenum. Edited by M Feldman. Philadelphia: Current Medicine LLC, 1996.

H_2-receptor antagonist or proton pump inhibitor for 8–12 weeks. With eradication of *H. pylori* and the cessation of NSAIDs, most ulcers do not recur. Sealed, uncomplicated perforations confirmed by contrast study can be managed conservatively with bowel rest and acid anti-secretory medication until the symptoms resolve.

Operative

Peptic ulcers are rarely seen in surgery today. Optimal management of complicated or non-healing ulcers requires surgical excision. Many operations also require an acid-reducing and gastric drainage procedure at the time of operation. Evidence of perforation, obstruction or persistent hemorrhage requires emergent operation, which is usually best achieved with a distal antrectomy and truncal vagotomy. Reconstruction may be achieved with either gastroduodenostomy or gastrojejunostomy. However, in practice these procedures are seldom carried out and a simple perforation is managed with laparoscopic sutures.

Chest X-ray showing a perforated peptic ulcer

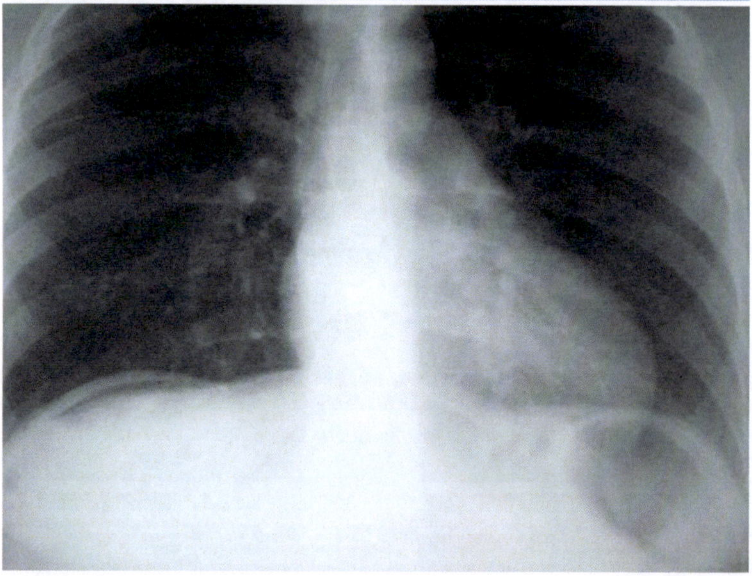

Figure 3.3 Chest X-ray showing a perforated peptic ulcer. Air is present under the right hemidiaphragm in a patient with acute severe abdominal pain. This patient had Zollinger–Ellison syndrome and a perforated anterior duodenal bulbar ulcer. From Wilcox C. Gastroenterology and hepatology: stomach and duodenum. Edited by M Feldman. Philadelphia: Current Medicine LLC, 1996.

Acute cholecystitis

Pathophysiology

Acute cholecystitis is the most common diagnosis in patients presenting with upper abdominal pain and fever. Inflammation of the gallbladder is most commonly caused by cholelithiasis (*see* Figure 3.4), where it develops in about 3% of patients. Cholelithiasis may also lead to obstruction of the cystic duct or common bile duct (Mirizzi syndrome). This obstruction leads to increased intra-luminal pressure in the gallbladder, which can result in localized inflammation, edema, and necrosis of the mucus wall. *Clostridium perfringens*, a gas-producing and causative bacteria of cholelithiasis, has a distinctive X-ray image with visible gas perforations, and can therefore be easily identified.

Medical history and physical examination

Patients with acute cholecystitis will commonly complain of right upper quadrant abdominal pain, which worsens several hours after oral intake of food.

Acute cholecystitis

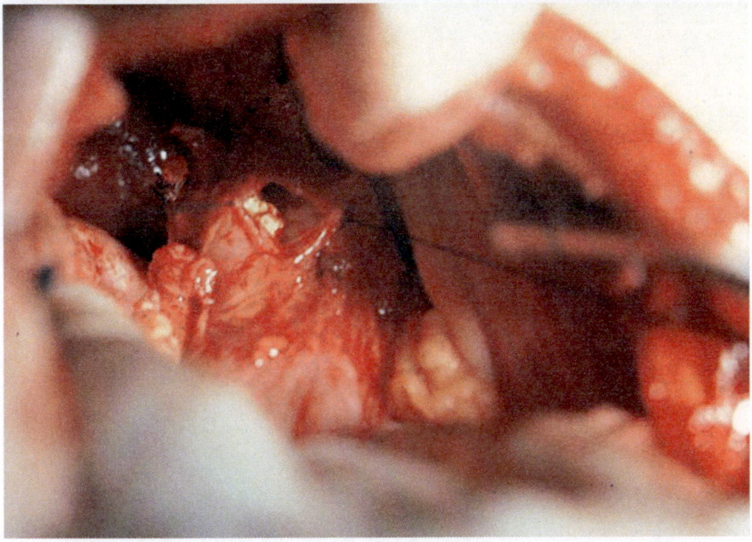

Figure 3.4 Acute cholecystitis. Operative view of patient shows the common bile duct stone and ascending cholangitis. From Finegold et al. Atlas of infectious diseases: intra-abdominal infections, hepatitis, and gastroenteritis. Edited by G Mandell, B Lorber. Philadelphia: Current Medicine LLC, 1997.

Murphy's sign (ie, the arrest of inhalation with deep right upper quadrant palpation) is highly suggestive of acute cholecystitis. A mild jaundice may accompany cholecystitis as a result of inflammation and edema surrounding the biliary tract.

Laboratory studies

While patients are likely to have a normal complete blood count and metabolic panel, liver function tests may be variably elevated due to cholestasis, with specific elevation of alkaline phosphatase. Among patients with acute cholecystitis, 50% will have bacterial organisms in their bile. This incidence increases with age to 80% in patients who are more than 80 years of age. In addition, 10% of patients with acute cholecystitis will have a bacterial infection comparable with acute appendicitis.

Diagnostic imaging

Ultrasound scanning is the imaging of choice in patients suspected of having acute cholecystitis (*see* Figure 3.5). Sonographic findings of peri-cholecystic fluid, a distended gallbladder wall and gallstones suggest acute cholecystitis, whereas ultrasonic Murphy's sign is nearly pathognomic. Equivocal circumstances may need biliary scintigraphy (hydroxy iminodiacetic acid [HIDA] scan) to make the definitive diagnosis.

Simple cholecystitis with gallstones

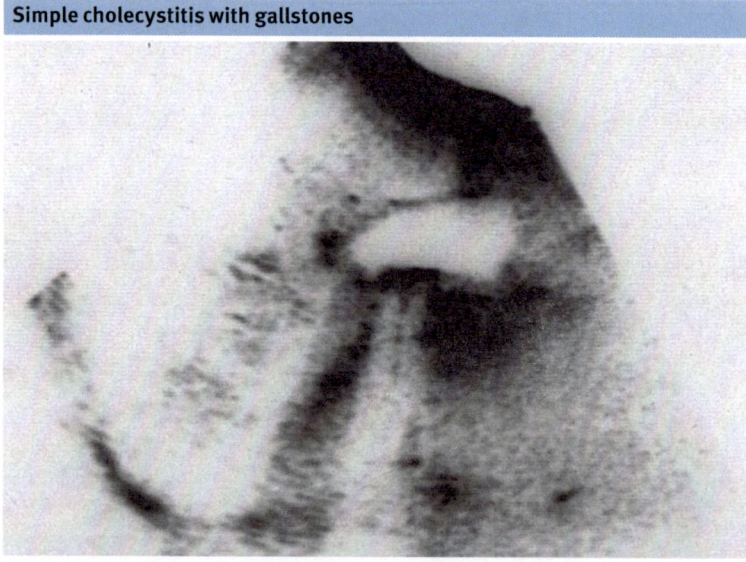

Figure 3.5 Simple cholecystitis with gallstones. In more than 90% of cases of acute cholecystitis, gallstones are impacted in the cystic duct. It is assumed that a sudden change in the degree of obstruction leads to a sudden increase in intraductal pressures, producing gallbladder distension and compromising blood supply and lymphatic drainage. This may proceed to necrosis of tissues and proliferation of bacteria. From Finegold et al. Atlas of infectious diseases: intra-abdominal infections, hepatitis, and gastroenteritis. Edited by G Mandell, B Lorber. Philadelphia: Current Medicine LLC, 1997.

Confirming the diagnosis

Patients with localized and continuous right upper quadrant abdominal pain together with sonographic findings are proven to have acute cholecystitis.

Resuscitation

Initial therapy consists of bowel rest, intravenous fluids, and pain control. Concerns about morphine contributing to sphincter of Oddi spasm have proven unwarranted. Since acute cholecystitis is acute inflammation, antibiotic administration is unnecessary. However, should elective cholecystectomy be chosen, single-dose antibiotic prophylaxis should be given at the start of the operation.

Interventional approaches

Non-operative

Most patients improve dramatically with bowel rest, intravenous hydration, and pain control.

Operative

In cases of acute cholecystitis where there is prolonged mechanical cystic duct obstruction, non-operative measures will be insufficient to treat the bacterial infection and any associated complications. In such cases, patients should undergo a cholecystectomy during the initial hospital admission. A more conservative approach (ie, with bowel rest, hyoscine, and tea, without any antibiotics), in dealing with most acute cholecystitis patients, has resulted in high mortality and complication rates in the past. Cholecystectomy after conservative treatment had a mortality rate of 16.7%, while early and late operations showed comparable results with mortality rates of 2.5–3.3% and 2.4%, respectively.

In cases of cholecystolithiasis, surgery is required. Given that today the risk of post-operative infection is very low, cholecystectomy should not be delayed, particularly as this may result in a potentially higher risk of post-operative bacterial complication. There is also a lower risk of morbidity when an operation is carried out early using a laparoscope. There are a number of arguments to support the trend toward early operation in acute cholecystitis, as summarized in Figure 3.6.

Complicated cholecystitis may require emergency surgery if generalized peritonitis or sepsis develop, although these patients may be better served by percutaneous cholecystostomy drainage, which results in an improvement in 75% of patients. A delayed cholecystectomy can then be performed when the patient's clinical condition improves; however, this is a technically more difficult procedure and can result in higher morbidity and mortality.

Reasons favoring early operation in acute cholecystitis
Clinical signs and symptoms
• Well characterized
Laboratory studies
• On average 50% of gallbladders with acute cholecystitis harbor organisms, which increases with age (eg, up to 80% in patients >80 years of age)
• As in cases of appendicitis, 10% of patients with acute cholecystitis have an infection
Diagnostic imaging
• Ultrasound shows stones in the gallbladder and often shows signs typical for acute cholecystitis (eg, edema sludge)
• Stones are often present combined with obstruction of the ductus–cysticus and edema

Figure 3.6 Reasons favoring early operation in acute cholecystitis

Acute cholangitis

Pathophysiology

Bile, while normally sterile, may become infected secondary to biliary obstruction and bacterial translocation from the gastrointestinal tract, usually the duodenum. Biliary instrumentation has become a significant secondary cause of cholangitis. In patients with jaundice and tumor obstruction, however, bile is always sterile, whereas in cases of gallstone obstruction (*see* Figure 3.7) there is an increase of biliary bacteria (bacteriobilia) to 50%, which continues to rise with age to bacterial counts consistently greater than 10^5/mL.

Gallstone obstruction in acute cholangitis

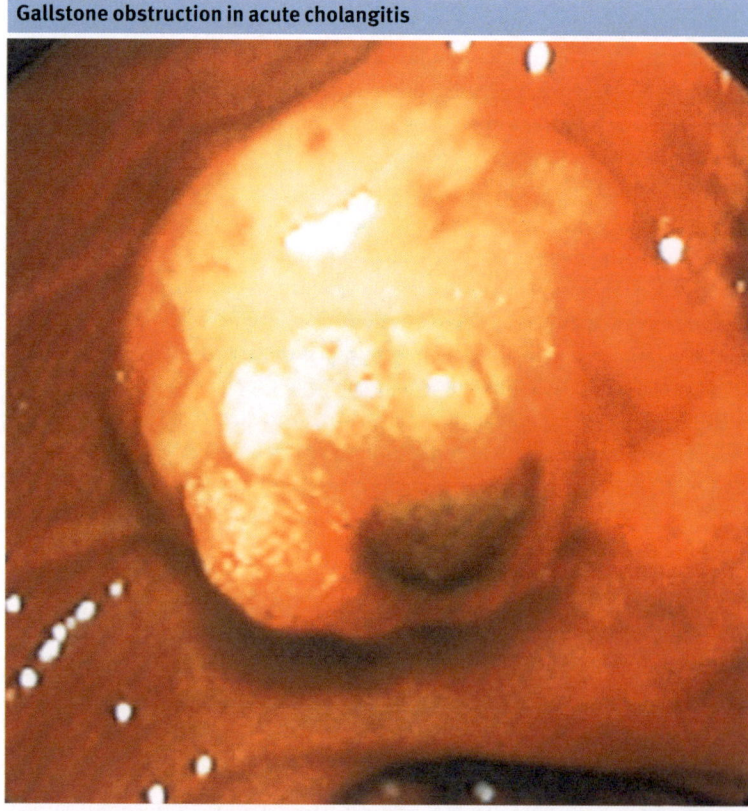

Figure 3.7 Gallstone obstruction in acute cholangitis. Stone disease remains the most common cause of cholangitis in most large series in the USA. Choledocholithiasis occurs in 8–15% of patients undergoing cholecystectomy; the incidence in patients more than 60 years of age is even higher, estimated at 15–60% in some series. At endoscopy, the obstructing stone is often seen bulging from the papillary orifice, as shown. From Davis et al. Gastroenterology and hepatology: gallbladder and bile ducts. Edited by M Feldman, NF LaRusso. Philadelphia: Current Medicine LLC, 1997.

Medical history and physical examination

The triad of jaundice, fever, and right upper quadrant abdominal pain described by Charcot, although classically taught, is rarely seen in clinical practice. Extreme cases of cholangitis may progress to mental obtundation and shock (Reynold's pentad). Most patients present with fevers of unknown origin, malaise, and vague abdominal pain.

Laboratory studies

Cholangitis leads to leukocytosis as well as an elevation in liver function tests – most notably, direct bilirubin and alkaline phosphatase. In addition, blood cultures will often be positive and confusion with hepatitis is possible in the early stages of the disease. Bile specimens can be obtained through the use of nasogastric tubes, or gastroscopes, that are inserted while carrying out endoscopic retrograde cholangiography (ERC).

Diagnostic imaging

The initial imaging to assess for cholangitis is abdominal ultrasound. Common bile duct dilation, gall bladder, or common bile duct stones and localized fluid collections are all evident on ultrasound. CT may be necessary if the diagnosis is in question or to plan therapeutic intervention. Endoscopic retrograde cholangio-pancreaticography (ERCP) should be attempted cautiously in the acute phase of cholangitis (see Figure 3.8). There are, however, exceptions in the case of very small stones where it is not unusual for the common bile duct to be undilated (such small stones are also often associated with acute pancreatitis); in the case of liver cirrhosis, the common bile duct also remains undilated.

Resuscitation

Initial therapy for cholangitis includes intravenous fluid administration and antibiotic therapy. Broad-spectrum antibiotic coverage should be initiated, with the addition of anaerobic coverage in patients who have had previous biliary instrumentation. Quinolones and broad-spectrum penicillins exhibit a high degree of biliary concentration.

Interventional approaches
Non-operative

The mainstay of intervention for cholangitis is non-operative in the form of ERCP or percutaneous trans-hepatic drainage of the obstructed biliary tree. During the acute phase of the disease, decompression of the biliary tree is the goal with definitive reconstruction or cholecystectomy at a later date.

Endoscopic retrograde cholangiopancreatography in acute cholangitis

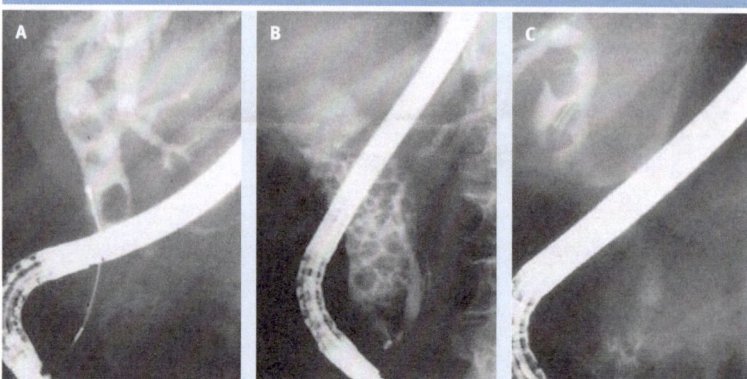

Figure 3.8 Endoscopic retrograde cholangiopancreatography in acute cholangitis.
Cholangiography is the gold standard for the diagnosis of choledocholithiasis. **A–C**,
Three examples of cholangiograms obtained by endoscopic retrograde cholangio
pancreatography. The choledocholiths are visualized as filling defects as a column of
contrast fills the common bile duct. Most stones that originate within the common bile
duct are brown pigment stones. Electron microscopy has revealed that such stones are
often associated with bacteria. Periampullary diverticula also seem to increase the risk
of choledocholith formation, perhaps by serving as a reservoir for intestinal bacteria. The
formation of a common bile duct stone around a surgical clip is shown in **C**. Foreign bodies,
including suture material placed 30 years before the patient presented with common bile
duct stones, have often been reported in association with choledocholithiasis. From Davis
et al. Gastroenterology and hepatology: gallbladder and bile ducts. Edited by M Feldman,
NF LaRusso. Philadelphia: Current Medicine LLC, 1997.

Operative

In patients unresponsive to non-operative drainage and antibiotic administration, emergent surgical drainage is warranted. Similar to percutaneous
drainage, the goal of operative drainage is to adequately drain the biliary tree
and reserve definitive therapy for when the patient recovers from the acute
illness. Decompression is necessary, but there is no reduction in bacteriobilia
with decompression alone, so antibiotics are also necessary as they only work
with bile flow.

Acute/complicated pancreatitis

Pathophysiology

There are several etiologies for acute pancreatitis; in industrialized society the
most common are choledocholithiasis and alcohol abuse. Other causes include
hypertriglyceridemia, hyperparathyroidism, malignancy, ERCP, and trauma.

This disorder varies markedly in severity and predictability. The majority of patients suffer mild attacks with spontaneous resolution and low mortality. In patients with complicated pancreatitis, adult respiratory distress syndrome, fluid sequestration, hepatic failure, pancreatic necrosis (*see* Figure 3.9), acute renal failure, and even death may ensue.

Medical history and physical examination
Patients may present with complaints of epigastric abdominal pain radiating around to the back like a belt, nausea and vomiting, acute jaundice, and varying degrees of systemic illness. A physical examination is generally unrevealing. Blue–gray discoloration of the flanks, due to exudation of fluid stained by pancreatic necrosis into the subcutaneous tissues, is known as Grey–Turner's sign. Similar discoloration in the peri-umbilical area is known as Cullen's sign. A fever on presentation is usually indicative of cytokine-mediated systemic inflammation.

Laboratory studies
Acute pancreatitis is confirmed with elevated serum amylase and lipase levels, although the degree of elevation does not correspond with disease severity. Lipase has a superior sensitivity and specificity for acute pancreatitis and is preferable to amylase for diagnosis. Other signs include significant base deficit, decreased hematocrit, elevated creatinine, and blood urea nitrogen reflecting volume contraction. The liver function test may also be elevated in cases of biliary obstruction from acute inflammation. Simple laboratory tests (eg, C-reactive protein, leukocyte) are also elevated.

Diagnostic imaging
Mild cases of pancreatitis with an unclear etiology require diagnostic imaging to establish a cause. Plain radiographs contribute little to the diagnosis; abdominal ultrasound is the standard imaging used to assess for cholelithiasis and acute cholecystitis. If no evidence of biliary disease is detected or in cases of severe pancreatitis, a CT scan (using contrast agents) of the abdomen is warranted to assess for fluid collections, phlegmon, abscess, and pancreatic necrosis (*see* Figure 3.10). The use of ERCP early on in the disease, in combination with sphincterotomy and ductal stone extraction, is gaining acceptance in the modern literature. It appears that this minimally invasive approach is warranted mainly in cases of acute pancreatitis, complicated by cholangitis and biliary sepsis.

Pathology of necrotizing pancreatitis

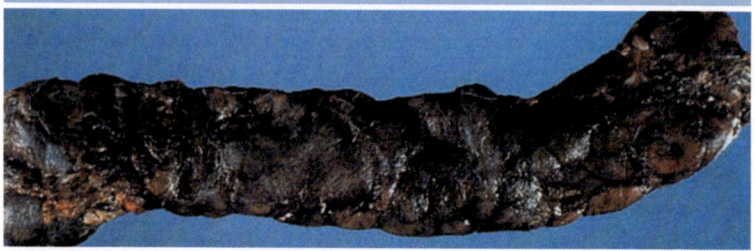

Figure 3.9 Pathology of necrotizing pancreatitis. Extensive ischemic–hemorrhagic necrosis is present in this gross pathology specimen. From Steinberg W. Gastroenterology and hepatology: pancreas. Edited by M Feldman, PP Toskes. Philadelphia: Current Medicine LLC, 1998.

Resuscitation

Mild pancreatitis simply requires intravenous hydration, bowel rest, and pain control, until the resolution of the episode. Early enteral feeding has been associated with improved outcomes. Severe pancreatitis may require admission to the intensive care unit with the above therapy plus nasogastric suction, enteral nutritional support (the nasojejunal route is recommended), cardiopulmonary support, and systemic antibiotics in some circumstances.

The use of antibiotics in pancreatitis continues to be debated; however, it is widely agreed that the use of antibiotic therapy is best reserved for treating cases of pancreatic necrosis and secondary infection. The use of prophylactic antibiotics is not widely supported in the modern literature.

Interventional approaches

Non-operative

There is a trend in the treatment of acute pancreatitis to adopt a more conservative approach and most cases of pancreatitis involve non-operative therapy. Cardiopulmonary support in conjunction with bowel rest is the mainstay of therapy for most cases of severe uncomplicated pancreatitis.

Operative

Today, there is much more discussion on how to classify patients with pancreatitis and when to start operative management. The greatest threat comes from pancreatic necrosis, which develops in 30–70% of cases depending on the literature cited, and accounts for 80% of deaths. The severity of a defined necrosis is measured using Ranson's criteria for acute pancreatitis. For patients

CT scan of the pancreas indicating gas bubbles within the substance of the pancreas

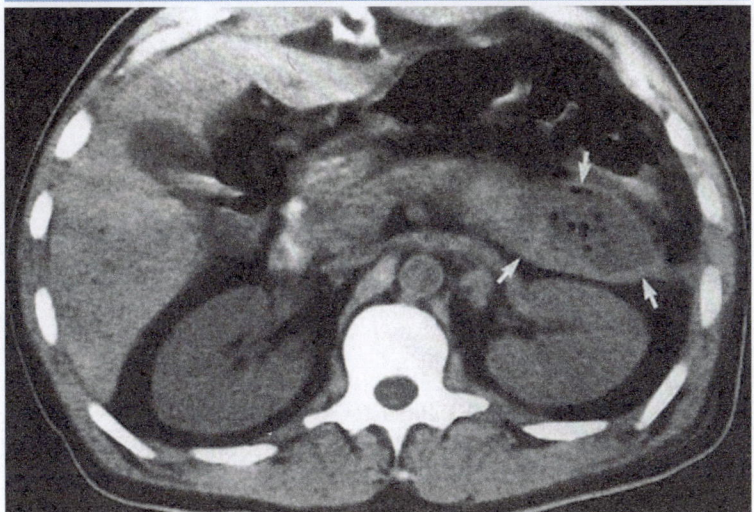

Figure 3.10 CT scan of the pancreas indicating gas bubbles within the substance of the pancreas. CT, computed tomography. The gas bubbles suggests a pancreatic abscess secondary to gas-producing organisms; however, sterile necrosis with microcommunication with the gut can lead to this CT finding. Only with a fine-needle aspirate can one diagnose an abscess with assurance. From Steinberg W. Gastroenterology and hepatology: pancreas. Edited by M Feldman, PP Toskes. Philadelphia: Current Medicine LLC, 1998.

with self-limited mild-to-moderate gallstone pancreatitis, a cholecystectomy should be undertaken during the initial hospital admission to prevent future episodes of pancreatitis.

Severe pancreatitis (eg, Ranson score >2.3) presents a very different situation; there is widespread agreement that surgical intervention is best avoided in nearly every case. The role of percutaneous drainage of peri-pancreatic fluid collections and abscesses is currently being explored in the literature. In patients with CT-proven necrosis lasting more than 2 weeks and with more than one organ failure, it is advisable to start antibiotic therapy. Only in severe cases of infected pancreatic necrosis and overwhelming sepsis, is exploratory laparotomy and pancreatic necrosectomy recommended. Early enteral feeding should also be considered to reduce the danger of recurrent infection and to restore normal bowel movement. These measures are basically important to stop antibiotic therapy, which is the next step to reduce further complication by organisms resistant to treatment.

In one prospective study by Robert (2002), early prediction of acute pancreatitis was not possible using serum markers, Ranson score, or even CT scan; ultimately, the decision concerning how and when to treat is a decision to be made by both the clinician and surgeon, who will base their choice on all available parameters.

Biliary pancreatitis

Immediate antibiotic treatment is mandatory for patients with biliary pancreatitis, even in mild cases. Between 50% and 80% of patients with acute cholecystitis or stone obstruction of the common bile duct will reveal 10^5 organisms per milliliter of bile. Stones are often very small and the choledochus cannot be seen distended in ultrasound. Small stones are more dangerous because they are difficult to detect. Decompression of the common bile tract by ERC alone does not reduce bacteriobilia; in this instance, antibiotics are indicated. Biliary excretion and the varying behavior of antibiotic agents in bile should also be considered; for example, tetracyclines and aminoglycoside are not effective in bile and modern penicillin (eg, acyl-aminopenicillin) is the only agent that is secreted even when bilirubin levels are extremely high. Bacteria can be eliminated within 24–48 hours. In these cases, early antibiotic treatment in combination with ERC or cholecystectomy, depending on the patient's condition and any comorbidities, is indicated.

Acute appendicitis

Pathophysiology

Luminal obstruction is a key initiating factor in the pathogenesis of appendicitis. Lymphoid hyperplasia is a frequent cause in children and young adults. In the older population, fecaliths, calculi and luminal fibrosis play a more prominent role. Obstruction of the lumen ultimately leads to appendiceal distension, vascular congestion, and mural necrosis with perforation. Bacterial invasion of the appendiceal wall follows vascular compromise. Perforation leads to phlegmon, abscesses, or free intraperitoneal spillage, resulting in diffuse peritonitis (*see* Figure 3.11).

Medical history and physical examination

Patients with appendicitis typically present with vague umbilical discomfort that intensifies and localizes to the right lower abdominal quadrant, at McBurney's point (*see* Figure 3.12). Nausea and vomiting following the onset of pain suggests appendicitis, while diarrhea is an inconsistent symptom.

Anorexia has historically been cited as a very reliable risk factor for acute appendicitis; those patients without anorexia should receive careful reconsideration of their diagnosis.

Intra-operative view of acute appendicitis with gangrene and perforation

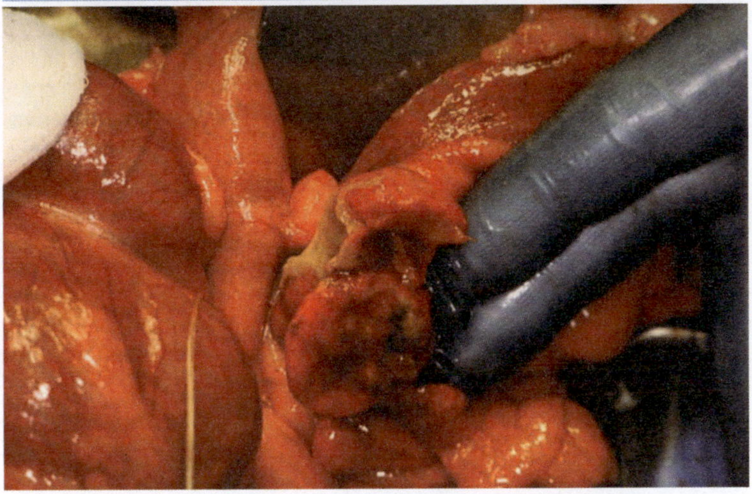

Figure 3.11 Intra-operative view of acute appendicitis with gangrene and perforation.

Laboratory studies

Patients will usually have an elevated leukocyte count with a left shift and a normal urinalysis; female patients should have pregnancy ruled out.

Diagnostic imaging

In equivocal cases, imaging is helpful to distinguish the pathologic cause of pain. Pelvic ultrasound is the first-line test in female patients with suspected gynecologic pathology, whereas appendicitis, diverticulitis and inflammatory bowel disease are best seen with abdominal CT (*see* Figure 3.13).

Confirming the diagnosis

While some cases of acute appendicitis are obvious, many present with enigmatic signs and symptoms. In these cases, the evaluating physician is faced with several options in order to determine the correct diagnosis, including:
- an abdominal CT;
- guarded observation with serial examinations; or
- diagnostic laparoscopy.

A review of 100 appendectomies carried out to find cases of acute appendicitis showed that the patients all presented with signs and symptoms of acute abdominal pain and tenderness in the lower quadrant of the abdomen, and all patients had ultrasound and laboratory test results, including a urine analysis. The intervention was always decided by the senior surgeon. The data showed that only 50% of the laboratory findings correlated with acute appendicitis. The usual characteristics and clinical signs (eg, pain, tenderness of the abdomen) and a thorough and repeated clinical assessment over time were the main factors given by the experienced surgeon to support the need for an operation. The diagnosis of acute appendicitis was right in 90% of cases. The correct diagnosis of appendicitis has yet to significantly improve either with more frequent use of diagnostic imaging techniques or by laboratory testing. The best tool in deciding when to operate remains the experienced surgeon.

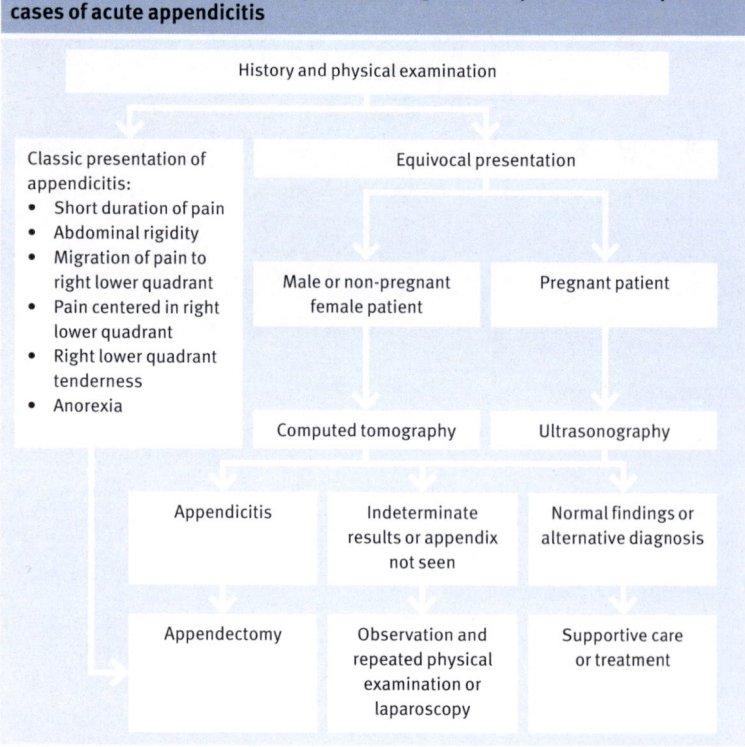

Figure 3.12 Algorithm for the evaluation of pain in the right lower quadrant in suspected cases of acute appendicitis. Reproduced with permission from Paulson et al. Suspected appendicitis. N Engl J Med 2003; 348:236–42 © Massachusetts Medical Society.

Resuscitation

Patients suspected of acute appendicitis should receive pre-operative intra-venous fluid resuscitation and intravenous antibiotics effective against polymicrobial intra-abdominal bacteria while they are being prepared for the operating room.

Interventional approaches

Acute appendicitis followed by appendectomy ensures that the source of infection is eradicated, and is therefore the basis for the best possible outcome. There are, however, some studies which seem to prove that antibiotic

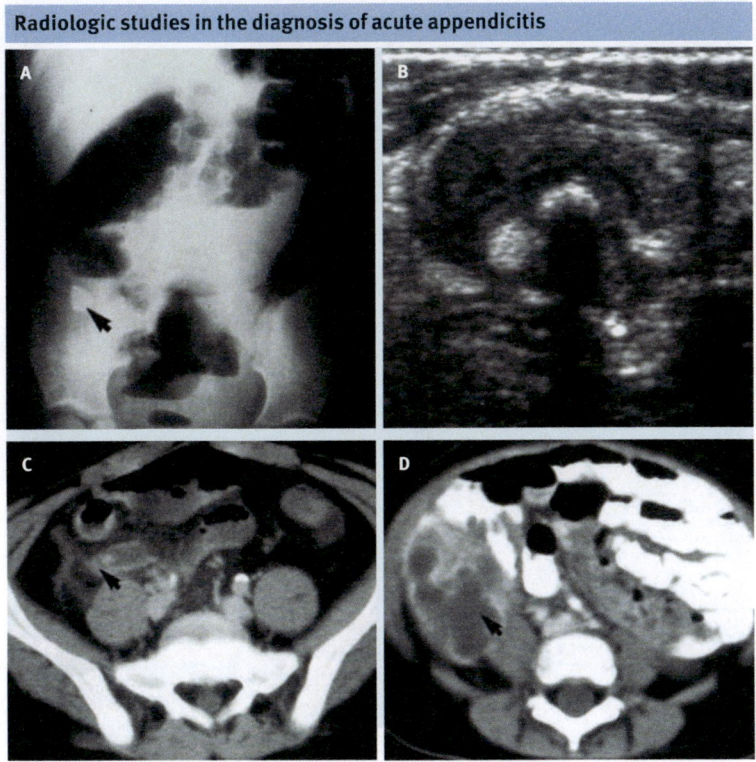

Radiologic studies in the diagnosis of acute appendicitis

Figure 3.13 Radiologic studies in the diagnosis of acute appendicitis. A, Abdominal radiograph showing appendicolith (arrow) and local ileus in lower abdomen. **B,** Ultrasound showing cross-section of a non-compressible, thick-walled tubular structure with acoustic shadowing from an appendicolith. **C,** CT scan showing thick-walled structure with surrounding inflammation in right lower abdomen (arrow). **D,** CT scan showing localized appendiceal abscess in right lower abdomen (arrow). From Langer J. Gastroenterology and hepatology: pediatric gastrointestinal problems. Edited by M Feldman, PE Hyman. Philadelphia: Current Medicine LLC, 1997.

treatment of appendicitis is a potential option. Randomized trials, however, have clearly defined inclusion and exclusion criteria, and are performed under somewhat artificial and controlled conditions. While this allows both known and unknown confounders to be controlled, findings from a randomized clinical trial cannot always be extrapolated to a patient population. In Europe, the operative approach is the procedure of choice in nearly all instances. The outcome of a randomized study can be speculated; new modern antibiotic agents will produce similar results in either case if the operation is carried out early or after conservative treatment. The only difference will be the longer treatment period for the patient and more interventions.

Non-perforated appendicitis

In cases of non-perforated appendicitis, open or laparoscopic appendectomy are advocated techniques. Laparoscopy is often preferred if the diagnosis is in question, if there is a concern for pelvic pathology, and in obese patients.

Perforated appendicitis

Patients with a CT-confirmed diagnosis of perforated appendicitis with associated abscess may be considered for percutaneous drainage if it is technically feasible. The treatment will focus on continued drainage and intravenous antibiotics. The need for interval appendectomy at 6 weeks, while traditionally advocated in some parts of the world, has recently become controversial and there is much debate concerning its use, particularly in Europe. Patients with perforated appendicitis without evidence of abscess should proceed to appendectomy. Patients with an abscess not amenable to percutaneous drainage should proceed to surgical drainage of the fluid collection and be considered for interval appendectomy.

Ischemic colitis

Pathophysiology

Acute abdominal pain caused by spontaneous ischemic colitis occurs without any demonstrable vessel occlusion on angiography; the presumption being that this entity is caused by decreased blood flow to the colon. The spectrum of disease varies from mild submucosal edema to frank full-thickness necrosis (*see* Figure 3.14). Most cases are of the milder self-limiting variety seen primarily in middle-aged and elderly patients.

Ischemic colitis

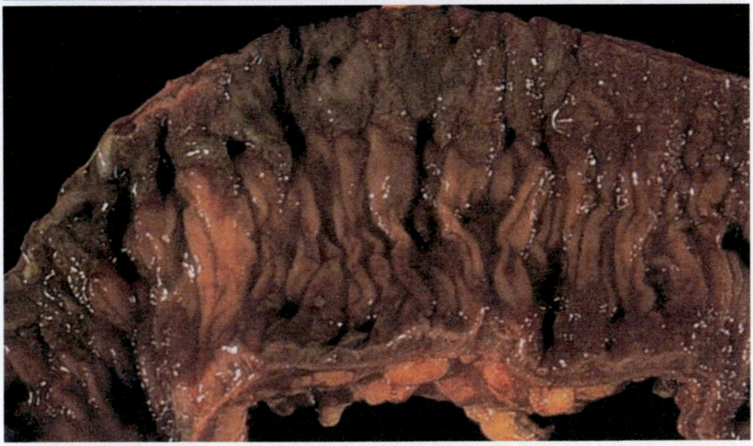

Figure 3.14 Ischemic colitis. Grossly, the mucosa is inflamed and hemorrhagic with scattered deep ulcers and a greenish pseudomembrane representing sloughed mucosa. From Friedman et al. Gastroenterology and hepatology: colon, rectum, and anus. Edited by M Feldman, CR Boland. Philadelphia: Current Medicine LLC, 1996.

Medical history and physical examination

Patients with spontaneous ischemic colitis typically present with a sudden onset of usually mild, cramping abdominal pain, mostly on the left side. Often, bloody diarrhea will accompany the pain within 24 hours. The left lower abdominal quadrant will be tender to palpation. Fever and tachycardia may also be present, and blood and slime may be present in feces.

Laboratory studies

Ischemic colitis may lead to anemia and leukocytosis. Necrosis of the colon may produce a profound acidemia, lactic acidosis, shock, and high temperature.

Diagnostic imaging

A diagnosis of ischemic colitis can be confirmed with endoscopy or a barium enema study. Endoscopy is preferred since it can be carried out at the bedside, and the colonic mucosa can be seen directly (*see* Figure 3.15). A barium enema will show a typical thumb-printing pattern, which results from submucosal edema and hemorrhage, but it is contraindicated if the patient has signs of peritonitis or sepsis, which increases the likelihood of full-thickness necrosis.

Resuscitation

Patients suspected of ischemic colitis should receive intravenous fluids and blood transfusions to replace any volume lost through bloody diarrhea. In addition, broad-spectrum antibiotics effective against colonic flora are essential to guard against the possibility of bacterial translocation from the ischemic colon.

Endoscopic appearance of ischemic colitis

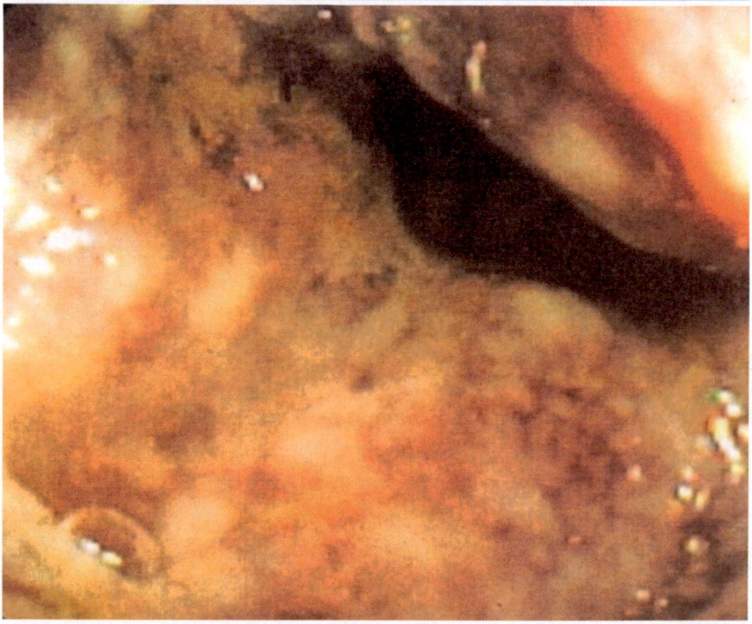

Figure 3.15 Endoscopic appearance of ischemic colitis. Ischemic colitis enters into the differential diagnosis of inflammatory bowel disease, particularly in elderly patients. The etiology is usually nonocclusive ischemic damage to the colon as a result of hypotension or hypoperfusion. Iatrogenic injury to, or ligation of, the inferior mesenteric artery may also result in ischemic colitis. The rectum is typically spared, colonic involvement is segmental, and the symptoms are acute and self-limited. Typical endoscopic features include ulceration, which is patchy and in severe cases, as shown here, associated with necrosis and exudation. In some cases, resolution may be followed by stricture formation. From Friedman et al. Gastroenterology and hepatology: colon, rectum, and anus. Edited by M Feldman, CR Boland. Philadelphia: Current Medicine LLC, 1996.

Interventional approaches

Operative

Rarely, patients may present with full-thickness necrosis from ischemic colitis or progress to necrosis and perforation during therapy. Any patient with signs of peritonitis or failing to improve with non-operative therapy requires an exploratory laparotomy and resection of the involved bowel. Primary anastomosis or diverting colostomy are options determined at the time of surgery based on the condition of the colon and the hemodynamic stability of the patient.

Non-operative

Most patients with ischemic colitis will improve with bowel rest, intravenous hydration and intravenous antibiotics, and usually there are no sequelae. Failure to improve may necessitate an operative approach, which involves resection of any non-viable colon and consideration of colostomy or primary anastomosis.

Diverticulitis

Pathophysiology

Colonic diverticula are an out-pouching from the colon wall, categorized as either true diverticula (containing all bowel wall layers) or false diverticula (containing only the mucosal layer) (see Figure 3.16). Diverticulosis is routinely used to describe a false diverticulum, most commonly located on the left side of the colon. Diverticula develop due to multiple factors, which include an inherent weakness in the colon wall where the vasa recta penetrate the colon along the border of taenia coli, a low fiber diet, and hard stools.

True diverticula of the colon are usually found in the cecum; however, 90% of colonic diverticula are located in the sigmoid colon. Colonic diverticulosis occurs in 5% of individuals at age 50 years and progresses to 80% of individuals at age 80 years. Diverticulitis is the inflammation and perforation of diverticula, often limited to a microscopic perforation. Symptomatic diverticulitis develops in 20% of individuals with diverticula.

Medical history and physical examination

Patients with diverticulitis usually present with left lower quadrant abdominal pain, tenderness, and involuntary guarding. In addition, non-specific gastrointestinal and urinary symptoms may also be present.

Laboratory studies

Patients commonly have an elevated leukocyte count and abnormal urinalysis.

Diagnostic imaging

An upright chest X-ray can be used to detect any free air in the peritoneal space. A barium enema and endoscopy should be avoided in the acute period of diverticulitis because of the risk of perforation. Ultrasound can be advantageous but is user-dependent and therefore of variable use. Abdominal CT is the gold standard for diagnosis of acute diverticulitis and the presence of any perforation or abscess (*see* Figure 3.17).

Diverticulitis of the colon

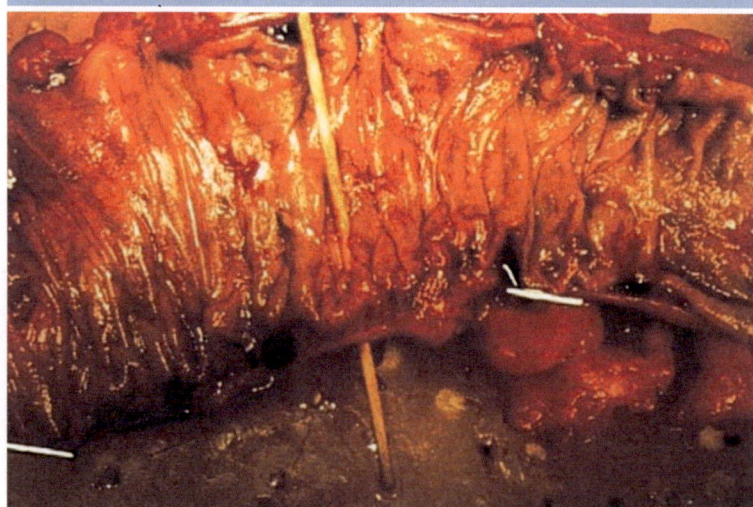

Figure 3.16 Diverticulitis of the colon. This operative specimen demonstrates that perforation usually occurs through an isolated diverticulum to create the clinical picture recognized as diverticulitis. Often such perforations will seal and heal completely. The probe has been passed through the site of the perforation. Note that the mucosal surface of the colon is otherwise normal, despite the presence of numerous diverticula. From Rothenberger et al. Gastroenterology and hepatology: colon, rectum, and anus. Edited by M Feldman, CR Boland. Philadelphia: Current Medicine LLC, 1996.

Confirming the diagnosis

During the acute phase of the disease, the diagnosis is often presumptive. Once the acute inflammation subsides, colonoscopy is recommended to confirm a diagnosis of diverticulosis and assess the extent of the disease, as well as to screen for possible malignancies.

Resuscitation

While no disease-specific resuscitation issues exist for diverticulitis, a severe episode may result in sepsis syndrome or septic shock. Fluid resuscitation and cardiopulmonary support should begin as soon as hemodynamic instability is recognized and include broad-spectrum antibiotics directed to intra-abdominal bacterial flora.

Multiple diverticula throughout the colon and sigmoid

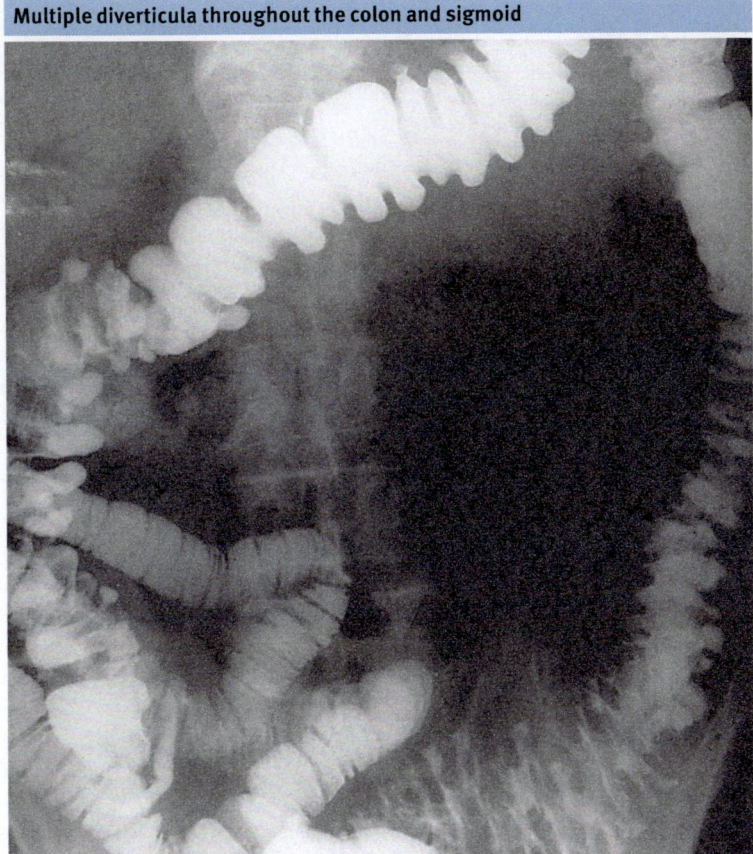

Figure 3.17 Multiple diverticula throughout the colon and sigmoid. A CT scan with oral and rectal contrast material is now the procedure of first choice, because CT scans are more sensitive than radiologic examinations and better demonstrate the extent and complications of diverticular inflammation. When diverticulitis is suspected but not found, the CT scan more often shows an alternative etiology for the signs and symptoms. The value of sonography in the work-up of diverticulitis is not yet established. From Finegold et al. Atlas of infectious diseases: intra-abdominal infections, hepatitis, and gastroenteritis. Edited by G Mandell, B Lorber. Philadelphia: Current Medicine LLC, 1997.

Uncomplicated diverticulitis

The first step in treating mild diverticulitis is bowel rest, without the use of antibiotics. If this is unsuccessful, treatment can be on an outpatient basis with broad-spectrum oral antibiotic coverage, with the caveat that diabetic and immunosuppressed patients should not be treated as outpatients due to the risk of overwhelming sepsis. Once the acute episode has resolved, screening colonoscopy and a high-fiber diet are recommended.

Complicated diverticulitis

Moderate or severe attacks of diverticulitis should be treated as an inpatient with intravenous broad-spectrum antibiotics, bowel rest, and pain control. Resolution of fever, correction of elevated white blood cell count and improvement of peritoneal signs determine resolution of the acute phase. In cases of complicated diverticulitis that do not resolve, intervention is warranted. The complications of diverticulitis include:

- *Abscess* – small peri-colic abscesses can be treated with antibiotic therapy only, however large abscesses require drainage. CT-guided drainage has become the treatment of choice for most abscesses. Fluid collections not amenable to percutaneous drainage may require surgical intervention to ensure adequate drainage. The timing of surgical drainage is determined by the patient's response to antibiotic therapy.
- *Obstruction* – obstruction can occur from inflammation. Resection of the inflamed region is mandatory (to rule out a tumor); however, if the obstruction resolves using conservative measures, the operation can be delayed to permit a bowel preparation and resolution of inflammation. In Europe, most surgeons do not believe that there is a need for mechanical bowel preparation. In the US, however, this is not the case as many surgeons still practice mechanical bowel preparation prior to colon surgery and parenterally administered antibiotics are used as prophylaxis alongside appropriate use of oral antibiotic bowel preparation.
- *Fistula* – fistula formation to adjacent structures may form from the colon to the bladder, vagina, small bowel, or skin. All require surgical repair consisting of resection of the involved colonic segment and primary repair of the adjacent organ. The timing of surgical intervention is usually delayed until the inflammation has subsided.

Initial diverticulitis

Most patients presenting with an initial episode of diverticulitis will resolve with medical therapy. Approximately a third of patients will resolve with no future symptoms, a third will continue to have vague abdominal complaints and a third will progress to a second episode of diverticulitis. Traditional teaching dictates that younger patients (<50 years) are offered an elective resection after an initial episode of complicated diverticulitis, due to the high recurrence rate over their remaining lifetime.

Recurrent diverticulitis

Since most patients presenting with a second episode of diverticulitis will develop one of the complications discussed above (ie, abscess, obstruction, or fistula), and 60% will develop a third episode, elective resection of the affected colon is recommended after the second episode for all patients.

Surgical intervention

Emergent resection

Emergent resection due to perforation, abscess, obstruction, or hemorrhage is usually a two-stage procedure (sigmoidectomy with end colostomy and closed rectal stump). For those patients who are hemodynamically unstable or unable to tolerate a full resection, a traditional two-stage procedure should be employed (diverting colostomy with resection of involved colon followed by reanastomosis when able). Even in these cases, it is possible to carry out primary resection and anastomosis to prevent further complications and restore normal bowel movement.

Elective resection

For patients undergoing an elective resection for symptomatic diverticulitis, a sigmoidectomy with primary colorectal anastomosis is the recommended procedure. It is not necessary to resect the entire colon with diverticula, only the segment of colon involved in the inflammatory response. Open, hand-assisted or entirely laparoscopic procedures are all equal options with comparable results.

Inflammatory bowel disease

Pathophysiology

While much has been made concerning the differences between the two kinds of inflammatory bowel disease (IBD), ulcerative colitis and Crohn's disease, the acute episodes of inflammation that occur with both diseases present with very similar symptoms (*see* Figure 3.18). Crohn's disease is a chronic relapsing transmural and segmental inflammatory disease, which may affect the entire gastrointestinal tract. Ulcerative colitis on the other hand, is a diffuse inflammatory disease limited to the mucosa of the colon and rectum.

Medical history and physical examination

Patients with either Crohn's disease or ulcerative colitis may present with abdominal pain, diarrhea, fever, weight loss, fatigue, or gastrointestinal bleeding with anemia. Both diseases are associated with extra-intestinal manifestations and Crohn's disease often involves anorectal lesions such as fissures, ulcers, or fistulas.

Ulcerative colitis and Crohn's disease

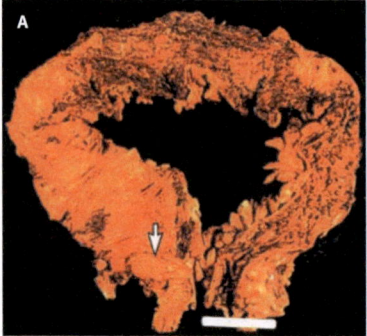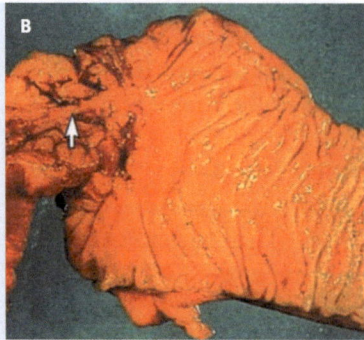

Figure 3.18 Ulcerative colitis and Crohn's disease. A, This total colectomy specimen shows a normal mucosal pattern in the terminal ileum and cecum (arrow) with diffuse involvement from the transverse colon to the rectum. The distal mucosa is erythematous and friable with many ulcers and erosions. **B,** This segment of colon shows a stricture in the right colon (arrow) with normal appearing mucosa in the distal portion of the specimen. Strictures in the right colon may be seen in both Crohn's disease and ischemic colitis. From Greenson J. Gastroenterology and hepatology: colon, rectum, and anus. Edited by M Feldman, CR Boland. Philadelphia: Current Medicine LLC, 1996.

Laboratory studies

There is no laboratory test to diagnose IBD, although a slight leukocytosis and mild anemia are often present. Other laboratory findings that may suggest IBD include an elevated erythrocyte sedimentation rate, increased levels of C-reactive protein, and hypoalbuminemia. Urinalysis is often normal.

Diagnostic imaging

While plain radiographs or contrast radiographs of the abdomen may suggest a diagnosis of IBD, the gold standard diagnostic tool is gastrointestinal endoscopy (*see* Figure 3.19). Friability and edema of the mucosa are clear signs of inflammation. The complications of IBD are often diagnosed with plain radiographs (free intraperitoneal air suggesting perforation), contrast radiography (thickened bowel wall suggesting mechanical obstruction), or CT (fluid collections or abscesses).

Confirming the diagnosis

Diagnosis of Crohn's disease or ulcerative colitis is confirmed by the presence of edema and chronic inflammation, whether transmural or mucosal, using endoscopic-directed biopsy.

An endoscopic view of severe Crohn's disease and ulcerative colitis

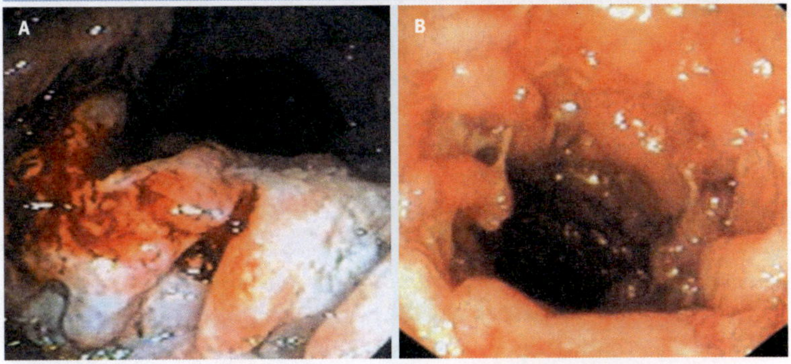

Figure 3.19 An endoscopic view of severe Crohn's disease and ulcerative colitis. A, Crohn's disease. Inflammatory bowel disease is a common cause of lower gastrointestinal bleeding in the younger patient. Patients with Crohn's disease usually present with abdominal pain and diarrhea but may have bleeding. Bleeding in inflammatory bowel disease is usually recurrent and minor. Profuse bleeding develops in up to 6% of patients with ulcerative colitis or Crohn's disease. B, Ulcerative colitis. The mucosa shows extensive ulceration and diffuse thickening with an inflammatory infiltrate. In contrast to Crohn's colitis, the ulceration lacks depth. From Friedman et al. Gastroenterology and hepatology: colon, rectum, and anus. Edited by M Feldman, CR Boland. Philadelphia: Current Medicine LLC, 1996.

Resuscitation

Patients with acute episodes of IBD are often anemic and dehydrated. Intravenous fluids and transfusion are often necessary. If these patients present with sepsis, broad-spectrum antibiotics targeted against colonic flora are indicated.

Interventional approaches
Non-operative

The goal of therapy is to alleviate symptoms, restore nutrition and subdue the inflammatory cascade. The main therapy for IBD is non-operative; acute episodes are treated with corticosteroids, while maintenance therapy is based on 5-amino-salicyclic acid (5-ASA) compounds administered either orally or rectally.

Operative

Surgical intervention for IBD is directed toward the complications of the disease process. The key complications include:

- *Toxic colitis* – with or without toxic megacolon, toxic colitis is an emergent life-threatening complication of IBD. Patients with toxic colitis present with fever, abrupt onset of bloody diarrhea, abdominal pain, and anorexia. Although rare, toxic colitis may be the initial presentation of patients with no prior history of IBD.

Initial treatment involves administration of intravenous fluids, intravenous broad-spectrum antibiotics, and bowel rest. Medical therapy is centered on 5-ASA compounds and steroids. Surgical intervention is necessary if patients with toxic colitis demonstrate evidence of free perforation, peritonitis, massive hemorrhage, or failure to improve within 48–72 hours of medical therapy. Surgical options include subtotal colectomy with end ileostomy (the best and first choice) or proctocolectomy with ileostomy (*see* Figure 3.20a).

- *Hemorrhage* – although rare, massive hemorrhage secondary to IBD requiring more than 6 units of blood in 24 hours usually requires surgical intervention. An upper gastrointestinal source of hemorrhage must be assessed prior to focusing on the lower gastrointestinal tract. Subtotal colectomy and end ileostomy remain the best options in ulcerative colitis. In Crohn's disease, which is often a segmental disease, it is important to localize the source of bleeding pre-operatively before proceeding to segmental resection. Localization options include endoscopy, angiography or 99m Tc-labeled red cell scan.

- *Perforation* – patients with intestinal perforation typically manifest significant abdominal or shoulder pain associated with fever and tachycardia. These patients usually require operative intervention. Perforation associated with ulcerative colitis necessitates a subtotal colectomy with end ileostomy. Treatment for perforation associated with Crohn's disease is tailored to the location of the gastrointestinal tract that is involved. Gastroduodenal perforations are best managed with debridement and primary repair. Jejunal–ileal perforations require resection and primary anastomosis if conditions are favorable. All other circumstances require resection of the involved bowel and diverting ileostomy.

- *Intra-abdominal mass or abscesses* – the majority of intra-abdominal abscesses associated with IBD are related to transmural ulceration of the diseased bowel as seen with Crohn's disease. Traditional teaching has recommended operative drainage for the management of these abscesses; however, improved radiologic techniques have resulted in the increased use of percutaneous drainage, leading to decreased morbidity and improved outcomes. If an abscess is associated with perforation, then operative intervention is mandated, requiring intestinal resection and fecal diversion (*see* Figure 3.20b).

- *Intestinal obstruction* – while obstruction may occur with either inflammatory disease (*see* Figure 3.21), it is more commonly associated with Crohn's disease, where it affects nearly 50% of patients. The initial management of IBD patients with suspected intestinal obstruction is: medical therapy, intravenous fluids, bowel rest, and 5-ASA compounds or steroid therapy. With this therapy and resolution of the acute inflammation, the majority of obstructions will resolve. In the rare circumstance in which

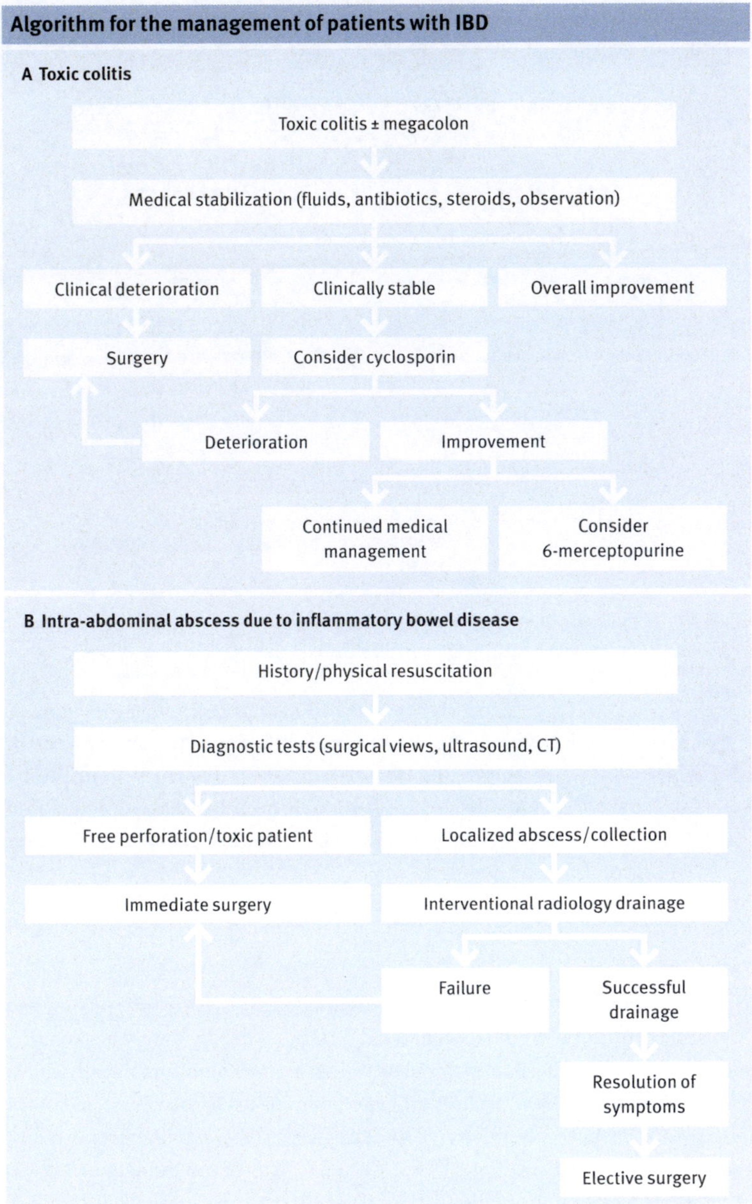

Algorithm for the management of patients with IBD

A Toxic colitis

Toxic colitis ± megacolon

↓

Medical stabilization (fluids, antibiotics, steroids, observation)

↓

Clinical deterioration	Clinically stable	Overall improvement

↓

Surgery	Consider cyclosporin

Deterioration	Improvement

Continued medical management	Consider 6-merceptopurine

B Intra-abdominal abscess due to inflammatory bowel disease

History/physical resuscitation

↓

Diagnostic tests (surgical views, ultrasound, CT)

↓

Free perforation/toxic patient	Localized abscess/collection

↓

Immediate surgery	Interventional radiology drainage

Failure	Successful drainage

Resolution of symptoms

↓

Elective surgery

Figure 3.20 Algorithm for the management of patients with IBD. CT, computed tomography. IBD, inflammatory bowel disease. Reproduced with permission from Berg et al. Acute surgical emergencies in inflammatory bowel disease. Am J Surgery 2002; 184:45–51 © Excerpta Medica, Inc.

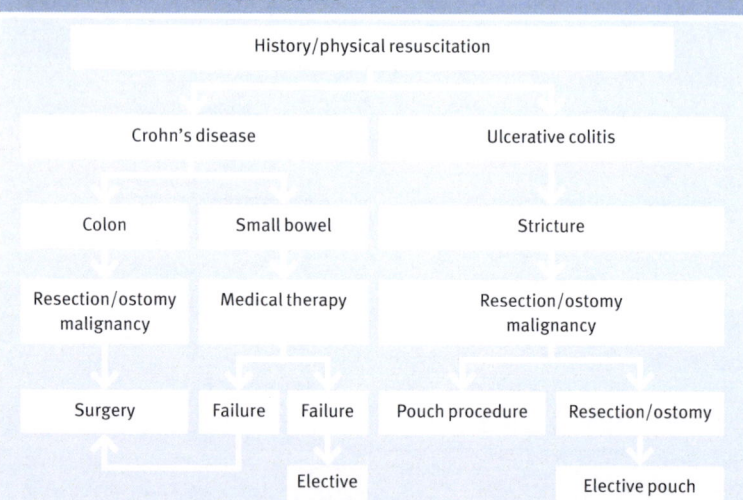

Algorithm for the management of patients with intestinal obstruction from Crohn's disease or ulcerative colitis

History/physical resuscitation

Crohn's disease

Ulcerative colitis

Colon

Small bowel

Stricture

Resection/ostomy malignancy

Medical therapy

Resection/ostomy malignancy

Surgery

Failure

Failure

Pouch procedure

Resection/ostomy

Elective surgery

Elective pouch procedure

Figure 3.21 Algorithm for the management of patients with intestinal obstruction from Crohn's disease or ulcerative colitis. Reproduced with permission from Berg et al. Acute surgical emergencies in inflammatory bowel disease. Am J Surgery 2002; 184:45–51 © Excerpta Medica, Inc.

the obstruction does not improve, operative intervention may be required. For patients with Crohn's disease, stricturoplasty has been found to be a safe and efficacious procedure for small bowel disease. For colonic Crohn's disease or ulcerative colitis, segmental resection with primary anastomosis is recommended.

Clostridium difficile colitis

Pathophysiology

The precipitating event for *Clostridium difficile* colitis is disturbance of the normal colonic flora. Broad-spectrum antibiotics, especially the cephalosporins and clindamycin, as well as overuse of proton pump inhibitors usually cause this disturbance and exacerbate *C. difficile*-associated diarrhea. New and more virulent strains have been detected and are associated with higher morbidity and mortality. When antibiotic therapy is administered for more than 3 days, the risk of developing antibiotic-associated diarrhea is more than doubled. Manifestations of the disease range from mild diarrhea to life-threatening *C. difficile* colitis.

C. difficile causes toxin-mediated colitis, expressed as two exotoxins: toxin A and toxin B. Although toxin A is more pathogenic *in vivo*, both toxins are responsible for an increase in inflammation, edema, and eventual focal ulceration of the colonic mucosa leading to transmural necrosis.

Medical history and physical examination
Patients with *C. difficile* colitis will present with a history of recent (up to the preceding 8 weeks) antibiotic use, abdominal pain, fever, and copious, often uncontrollable, diarrhea.

Laboratory studies
The *C. difficile* toxin can cause a profound leukocytosis (30,000–50,000/mm^3). The toxin is detectable using an enzyme immunoassay, although the gold standard is the cytotoxin assay.

Diagnostic imaging
Flexible sigmoidoscopy provides an immediate diagnosis; pseudomembranes located on the colonic wall are pathognomic for *C. difficile* colitis. CT findings of ascites, colonic wall thickening and colonic dilation also suggest infectious colitis (*see* Figure 3.22).

Resuscitation
Nearly all patients with *C. difficile* colitis are dehydrated from diarrhea with associated disturbances in electrolytes. Initial therapy consists of discontinuing the precipitating antibiotic and administering intravenous fluid hydration.

Interventional approaches
Operative
C. difficile colitis can progress to toxic megacolon or perforation with signs of sepsis and resistance to medical therapy. Operative therapy in this circumstance involves subtotal colectomy with end ileostomy and delayed reanastomosis.

Non-operative
First-line therapy consists of oral metronidazole administered three- or four-times daily (*see* Figure 3.23). However, metronidazole as a primary treatment option can fail or result in early recurrence. Alternative therapy is oral vancomycin (4 x 125 mg/day) which should be indicated especially in severe cases; intravenous vancomycin (same as oral dosage) is another alternative if oral medications are not tolerated.

CT scan of a patient with *Clostridium difficile* colitis

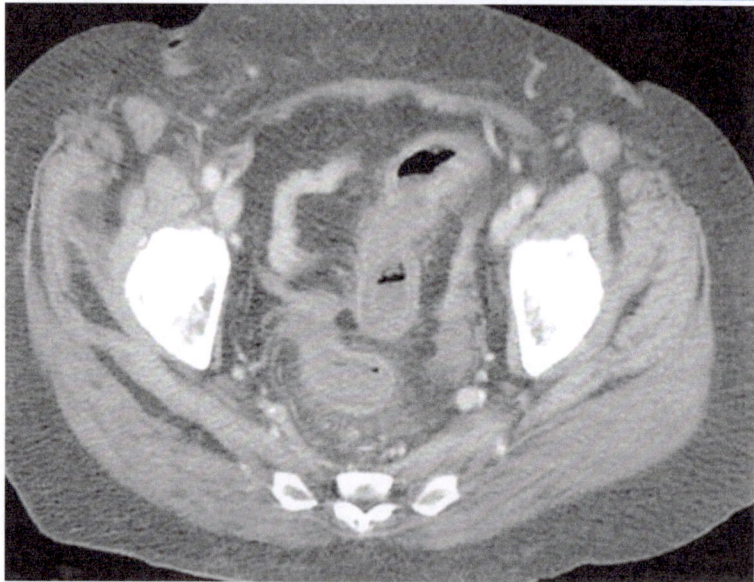

Figure 3.22 CT scan of a patient with *Clostridium difficile* colitis. CT, computed tomography. Abdominal axial CT view of a patient with *C. difficile* colitis demonstrating diffuse wall thickening of the rectum and sigmoid colon. Wall thickening is the key CT finding in *C. difficile* colitis. From Moyenuddin et al. Clostridium difficile-associated diarrhea: current strategies for diagnosis and therapy. Curr Gastroenterol Rep 2002; 4:279–286 © Current Science, Inc.

Post-operative intra-abdominal processes

Pathophysiology

Peritonitis or abscess presenting in the post-operative period is a complication of concern to most surgeons. Several situations are associated with a higher risk for the development of these complications, including operations performed in emergency settings or in less than ideal circumstances. Similarly, patients with significant comorbid conditions or malnutrition are also at increased risk. Causes include enteral spillage due to disease or during operation, anastomotic leakage due to technical errors, poorly healing tissues, or concurrent infection, which can lead to peritoneal seeding, tissue necrosis, or recurrent infection following surgical and antibiotic treatment (ie, tertiary peritonitis). These situations are often complicated by multi-resistant organisms and *Candida* spp. infections.

Medical history and physical examination

Suspicion of post-operative intra-abdominal infection is raised by the presence of a post-operative ileus, abdominal distention, fever, leukocytosis, intolerance of enteral feeding and organ failure (*see* Figure 3.24).

Laboratory studies

The most revealing laboratory finding for post-operative intra-abdominal complication is persistent leukocytosis. Other findings that support this diagnosis are anemia without a bleeding source, poor nutritional parameters, and moderate renal dysfunction. The risk of ongoing post-operative infection following secondary peritonitis and reoperation are high. Clinical predictive factors include age, comorbidities, the extent of contamination during the previous operation, inability to eliminate the cause of the primary disease, and pathological post-operative variables (eg, bilirubin, creatinine, lactate, PaO_2/FiO_2 ratio, albumin).

Diagnostic imaging

Imaging in the immediate post-operative period may be unrevealing; however, an abdominal ultrasound or CT scan 5–7 days post-operation may reveal a build-up of intra-abdominal fluid, suggesting the presence of an abscess or anastomotic leak.

Confirming the diagnosis

Signs of post-operative infection and findings on ultrasound or CT, make the diagnosis almost absolute. However, when no intra-abdominal findings are present other causes of post-operative fever, leukocytosis and failure to thrive must be considered. These other causes include pneumonia, urinary tract infections or acalculous cholecystitis, among others.

Resuscitation

The initial treatment for suspected intra-abdominal infection following an operation includes bowel rest, intravenous fluids, and early intravenous antibiotic therapy. The latter should be empirically based on the suspected contaminant from the operative site or organ (*see* Chapter 4).

Interventional approaches

Non-operative

It is important that post-operative intra-abdominal fluid collections, which are amenable to percutaneous radiographically guided drainage, should be drained promptly. Bacterial and fungal cultures should then be obtained from any fluid drained in order to guide antibiotic therapy.

Algorithm for the treatment of *Clostridium difficile*-associated diarrhea

Patient with suspected *C. difficile*-associated diarrhea

Diarrhea with one or more of the following:
- Recent antibiotic therapy
- Advanced age
- Multiple or severe comorbid diseases
- Nursing home resident
- Prolonged hospital stay
- Admission to intensive care unit

- Sharing of hospital room with *C. difficile*-infected patient
- Placement of nasogastric tube
- Use of antacids
- History of *C. difficile*-associated diarrhea

Physical examination findings:
- Acute abdomen (possible presentation)
- Fever
- Hypotension (occasionally)

Laboratory and imaging findings:
- Leukocytosis
- Dilation of colon on abdominal radiograph

- Perform stool studies to confirm *C. difficile* infection
- Correct fluid and electrolyte imbalance
- Provide cohort nursing and isolation if patient is hospitalized
- Start metronidazole

Able to stop antibiotics?

Yes

No

Resolved

Not resolved within 48 hours

Stable?

Yes

No

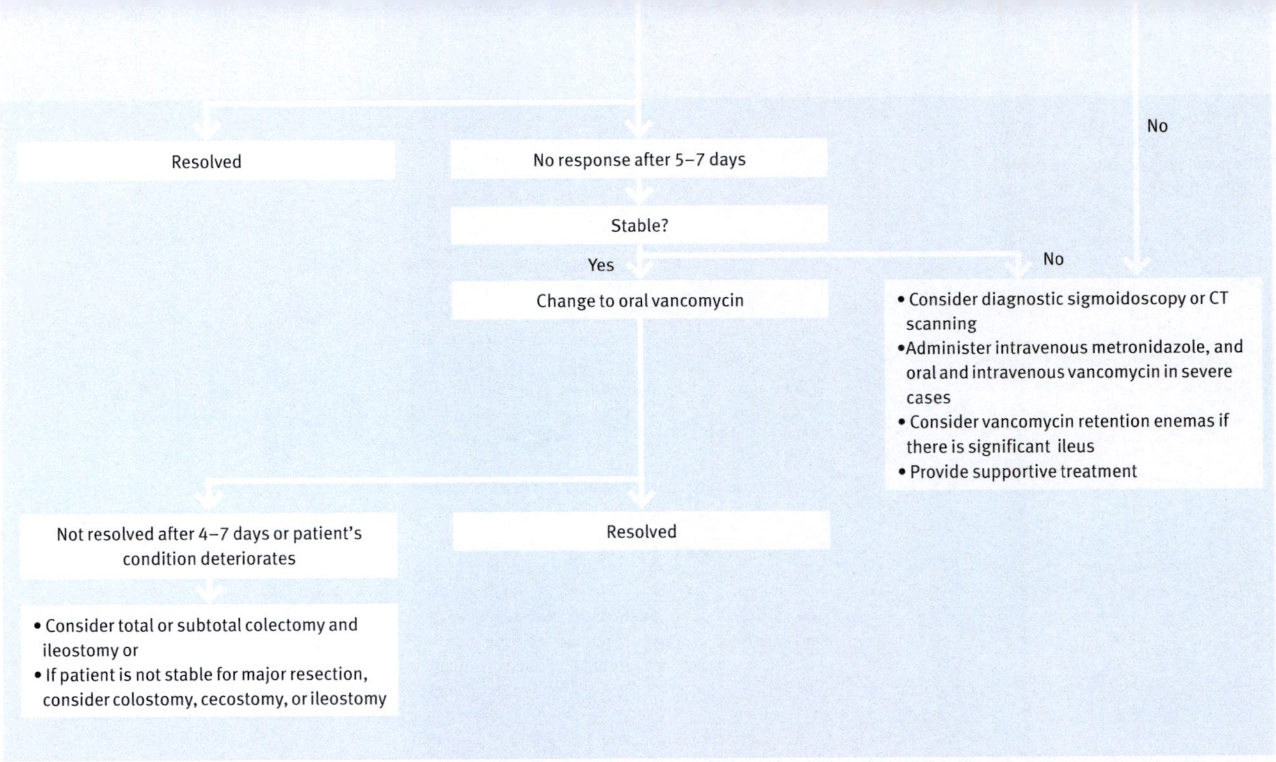

No

No

Resolved

No response after 5–7 days

Stable?

Yes

Change to oral vancomycin

Resolved

Not resolved after 4–7 days or patient's condition deteriorates

- Consider diagnostic sigmoidoscopy or CT scanning
- Administer intravenous metronidazole, and oral and intravenous vancomycin in severe cases
- Consider vancomycin retention enemas if there is significant ileus
- Provide supportive treatment

- Consider total or subtotal colectomy and ileostomy or
- If patient is not stable for major resection, consider colostomy, cecostomy, or ileostomy

Figure 3.23 Algorithm for the treatment of *Clostridium difficile*-associated diarrhea. CT, computed tomography. Reproduced with permission from Schroeder MS. Clostridium difficile-associated diarrhea. Am Fam Physician 2005; 71: 921–928 © American Academy of Family Physicians.

Algorithm for patients with postoperative intra-abdominal infection

Suspected intra-abdominal infection (post-surgical)

Please select:
- Ileus
- Distension and/or tenderness
- Recent intra-abdominal operation <5 days previously
- Recent intra-abdominal operation >5 days previously
- None of the above

1 and/or 2, None

1 and/or 2 and 3

- Consider re-exploration
- Consider other suspected causes

None

Does the patient have:
- Abdominal distension and evidence of organ failure?
- None of the above

Yes

1 and/or 2 and 4

Is the patient's bladder pressure:
- >20 cm H_2O?
- <20 cm H_2O?

<20 cm H_2O

>20 cm H_2O

Begin empiric antimicrobial therapy

Next

Undertake laparotomy and achieve adequate source control

- Terminate, continue or change antimicrobial therapy based upon operative findings
- When culture and susceptibility data are available, adjust antimicrobial therapy to treat identified pathogens

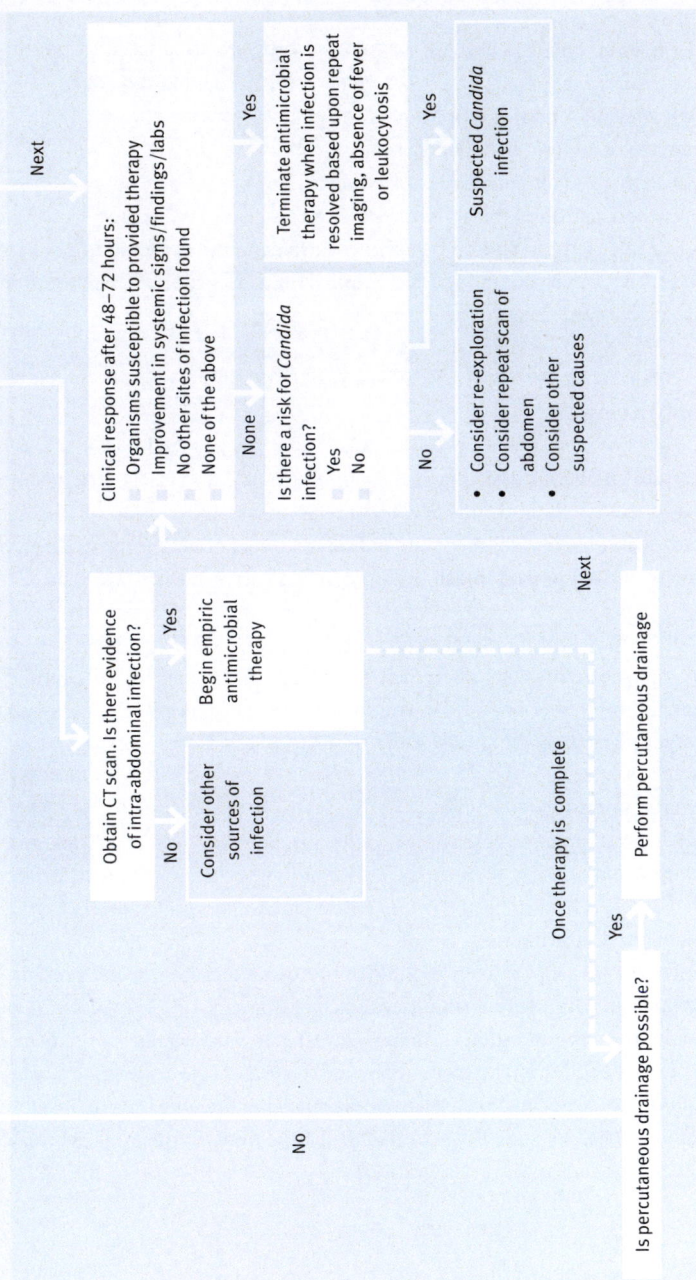

Figure 3.24 Algorithm for patients with postoperative intra-abdominal infection. CT, computed tomography.

Operative

In rare situations where percutaneous drainage is dangerous or not possible, it is then necessary to reoperate. The basic principles that should be adhered to are:

- complete abdominal exploration;
- drainage of all fluid collections;
- debridement of all necrotic tissue; and
- copious irrigation of the abdominal cavity.

Operative intervention should be carried out during the early post-operative period (<5 days post-operation) due to poor fluid collection and maturation of adhesive inflammation.

Post-operative superficial wound infection

Pathophysiology

The majority of post-operative wound infections are superficial and involve the skin and subcutaneous tissues superficial to the muscle and fascia. Risk factors for post-operative wound infection include advanced age, comorbid diseases (diabetes, malnutrition, etc), smoking, and length of operation. The most common pathogens causing wound infections are skin flora gram-positive bacteria.

Medical history and physical examination

This complication presents as erythema, drainage of serous or purulent fluid, fluctuance, and tenderness of the wound. Patients may complain of pain, tenderness, erythema, swelling or warmth of the incision.

Diagnostic imaging

Usually, wound infections are clinically obvious; however, ultrasound imaging may be helpful to clearly identify the extent of fluid collections and abscesses.

Interventional approaches

Treatment for post-operative wound infection is determined by the presence of fluctuance or drainage. Without evidence of drainage or a fluid collection, the treatment is simply antibiotic therapy directed toward the likely organism – gram-positive bacteria. With evidence of fluid collected under the skin, therapy (in addition to organism-directed antibiotics) includes opening the skin incision and draining the collected fluid. Inspection of the underlying fascia is crucial to assess for fascial infection or dehiscence.

Chapter 4

Antimicrobial management

Introduction

The term 'antibacterial chemotherapy' was first coined by the Nobelist Paul Ehrlich in 1906. According to Ehrlich, chemotherapy meant strictly treating bacterial infections without involving any immunological mechanisms and without disturbing organ function. Today, all classes of agents, developed synthetically or derived from nature (eg, bacteria, plant or fungi), are called antibiotics and work by directly killing bacteria or inhibiting bacterial growth. *In vivo* they also stimulate or inhibit innate immunoreactions. Immunomodulation by antibiotic agents is an area currently being researched to determine the true synergistic effects of antibiotic agents in treating bacterial infections.

Optimal use of an antimicrobial agent requires precise knowledge of a number of factors that the physician must carefully consider. These include:

- an understanding of the bacteriology of intra-abdominal infections, including the antimicrobial susceptibilities of the pathogen involved, its pharmacology and potential side effects;
- existing clinical data; and
- the origin of infection, time to surgery, source control and post-operative organ function.

Bacteriology of intra-abdominal infections

All cases of intra-abdominal infection result from organisms native to the gastrointestinal tract. There are more than 400 species of microorganisms, varying in type and concentration, that colonize the human gastrointestinal tract. The standard flora species is relatively identical, yet the composition varies between individuals. In a healthy state, the bacterial count in the stomach and small intestine is remarkably low, averaging 100 microbes/mL of both facultative and obligate anaerobic species. The number of bacteria, however, increases significantly if the acidity and motility of the gastrointestinal tract changes. In a healthy individual the gastric juice in the stomach contains low numbers of bacteria; the predominant species are *Streptococcus*, *Peptostreptococcus*, *Bacteroides*, gram-negative bacteria, and fungi. However, when the number of bacteria increases, *Candida* spp., for example, can be found in up to 60% of the gastric aspirate. Bacteria can also enter the stomach and intestine through contaminated meals, such as *Pseudomonas* spp. in tomato salad.

The predominant species in the ileum and colon are the same – *Enterobacteriaceae*, *Bacteroides fragilis* – and the colony counts are 10^6–10^8/mL. In our experience, bacterial counts in the peritoneal fluid of patients with gastric perforation are low in the first few hours after perforation but increase continually with time, and about 25% of the abdominal swabs taken were negative. Most organisms tend to be found as mixed flora (85%); however, *E. coli* and *B. fragilis* are the predominant species present. Bacterial counts are higher in the distal gastrointestinal tract, with numbers of mixed flora and bacterial counts being highest in cases of appendicular perforation. In the presence of infection, the pH is less than 7.0; if the peritoneal fluid is sterile or the bacterial count is low, the pH is greater than 7.0.

Looking at the sizeable literature on complicated intra-abdominal infection (ie, those infections requiring surgery or surgical intervention), it is evident that the same types of organisms continue to be reported over the years, as in the case of secondary peritonitis (*see* Figure 4.1). However, despite having a continual presence over the years, these organisms have failed to develop any major resistance to antibiotics, and can still be successfully treated with antimicrobial therapy.

Organisms reported to cause secondary peritonitis			
Organism	PEG 1987	USA 1995	Europe 1999
Escherichia coli	142 (58.0%)	375 (57%)	97 (51.3%)
Bacteroides fragilis	74 (30%)	249 (38%)	47 (24.9%)
Enterococcus spp.	65 (27%)	145 (22%)	56 (29.6%)
Streptococcus spp.	59 (25.2%)	226 (35%)	38 (20.1%)
Clostridium spp.	29 (12%)	102 (16%)	8 (4.2%)
Klebsiella spp.	28 (12.2%)	70 (11%)	15 (9.9%)
Candida spp.	23 (9.5%)	NK	14 (7.4%)
Pseudomonas aeruginosa	10 (4.1%)	63 (10.0%)	22 (11.6%)
Staphylococcus spp.	14 (5.8%)	63 (10.0%)	10 (5.3%)

Figure 4.1 **Organisms reported to cause secondary peritonitis.** NK, not known; PEG, Paul–Erhlich Foundation for Chemotherapy. Data from Wacha et al. Risk factors associated with intrabdominal infections: a prospective multicenter study. Langenbecks Arch Surg 1999; 384:24–32.

Antimicrobial susceptibility and resistance

Susceptibility testing

Susceptibility testing is used to determine the likely success of antibiotic therapy in a patient. There are a number of ways to test for antimicrobial susceptibility, and semi-automated methods are increasingly being used in practice. The testing is done *in vitro* whereby the growth response of the bacteria to an antibiotic is measured. Antibiotics that are shown initially to inhibit the growth of an organism are tested further; the antibiotic is diluted and different concentrations of the drug are placed in separate test tubes. A small amount of the test bacteria is then added to each test tube and, after inoculation, the minimum inhibitory concentration (MIC) level is identified. This is the lowest dose of a drug that prevents any visible growth of the inoculated organism. While the MIC level of a drug shows the dose that will prevent growth of the organism, this is not necessarily the dose that will kill the organism. By subculturing the contents of the 'no growth' test tubes to a solid medium, it is possible to determine the lowest concentration of the drug that actually kills the bacteria; this is known as the minimum bactericidal concentration (MBC).

While these results are extremely useful, they are not in themselves enough to choose the right agent for therapy and it is also important to consider the following:

- resistance patterns differ between geographical regions;
- MIC is measured at counts around 10^5/mL on agar plates; and
- temperature and pH are all standardized in a clinical setting.

Clinical reports of susceptibility and periodic summaries of antimicrobial susceptibilities of organisms from a hospital or institute are of considerable value. The results of antimicrobial testing are normally available 24–48 hours after the operation. Nonetheless, there are new intelligent automated methods, which, although not yet readily available in day-to-day practice, promise results 3–4 hours post operation. In reality, the decision concerning which agents to use should be made on the basis of past empirical evidence.

Resistance and underdosing

Resistance, which can depend on the levels of antibiotics in individual tissues, can be a consequence of underdosing, which may result in a considerably higher bacterial load (ie, $>10^8$/mL) in the tissues. Temperature, oxygen pressure, and pH value are also affected; this, in turn, may reduce the effectiveness of antibiotics in treating bacterial infections, as these agents perform best under normal homeostatic conditions.

Catecholamine therapy reduces intestinal organ perfusion and can lead to oxygen reduction, which significantly reduces the efficacy of quinolones. Catecholamines, such as arterenol, dobutamine, and dopexamine, can also increase perfusion in the splanchnic area. Obligate anaerobes produce acids that lower the pH of the intestine to 7.4 or less, thus making the use of amino glycosides ineffective for treatment.

In vitro results do not consider the pharmaco-kinetic (PK) and -dynamic (PD) effects of a given agent. Recently proposed PK and PD models have tried to assimilate all possible organ functions into a whole body model in order to simulate the clinical situation.

Using an animal model, it was possible to show two different effects depending on the agent being used, namely that:

- The activity of β-lactam antibiotics, vancomycin, macrolides and clindamycin are time dependent.
- The effectiveness of aminoglycosides and quinolones correlate with the concentration administered.

These differences partly explain the inferior results achieved with aminoglycoside in earlier studies. Since the 1990s, prospective randomized studies have shown that low doses of aminoglycosides are less efficacious than newer comparators. In one study, Solomkin et al. (1990) compared imipenem/cilastin to the gold standard of tobramycin/clindamycin, and the former proved to be more effective than the latter in improving outcome at the site of intra-abdominal infection. Bailey et al. (2002) carried out a meta-analysis more than a decade later, which showed similar results.

It is customary to look at the MIC as a parameter for the effectiveness of a therapeutic agent; however, considering the development of resistance a much higher dosage has to be administered – the so-called mutant prevention concentration (MPC). For example, as the concentration of fluoroquinolone increases, the proportion of organisms recovered initially falls dramatically.

Even with short-term (ie, one or two doses) antibiotic use, resistant organisms can be detected immediately. More than 70% of wound infections after prophylaxis are due to antibiotic-resistant bacteria. Multi-resistant organisms are found even after a short course of antibiotic treatment and more so after prolonged prescription of antibiotics. In the case of 'prophylactic antibiotics' in the treatment of pancreatitis, the impact on the residential flora of the gut is considerable and even a single dose of some antibiotics can lead to *C. difficile* selection. Past studies have shown that there is effective reduction of some bacterial strains in the gut, following oral intake of antibiotics after 3–5 days, whereas other strains continue to increase over the same time period. Continuing the regimen does not mean a complete and persistent eradication; some organisms are found to be in exactly the same numbers 8–10 days after treatment as they were prior to initiation of antibiotic therapy. These studies therefore show that for an antimicrobial agent to be effective, it must be administered in the maximum concentration possible.

Clinical studies
Early pre-clinical studies
Early animal studies form the basis of our understanding of how to treat intra-abdominal infections. In one study, an animal model of colonic perforation was used to examine the efficacy of 29 antimicrobial regimens in the treatment of intra-abdominal sepsis. Efficacy was judged on mortality during the first 12 days after antibiotic administration, and on the incidence of intra-abdominal abscesses noted at necropsy upon completion of the experiment. Antimicrobial agents active against *E. coli* prevented early mortality, whereas drugs active against *B. fragilis* were effective in reducing abscess formation. In this experiment, metronidazole produced a significant reduction in mortality, and chloramphenicol was shown to cause only a modest reduction in abscess formation. Optimal results were obtained with several regimens that show good *in vitro* activity against both coliforms and *B. fragilis*.

These animal experiments have shown that the number of *E. coli* in the peritoneal fluid correlated with mortality, whereas obligate anaerobes correlated with abscess formation. Administration of the most appropriate antibiotic agent resulted in lower mortality rates or minor abscess formation. Finding an agent, or a combination of agents, effective against both anaerobic and aerobic organisms seems to be the solution. In clinical practice, however, only a few antibiotics (eg, imipenem, moxifloxacin) are effective against both types of organism and these are discussed later in this chapter.

Clinical trials
Most clinical trials, especially those concerning complicated intra-abdominal infection, are designed to prove that a new therapy has equivalent, if not better, efficacy and tolerance as the standard therapy. According to the inclusion and exclusion criteria for most clinical trials, selected cases are at a minor risk for both complications and mortality. However, in prospective unselected collectives, the mortality of diffuse peritonitis, for example, is estimated to be 47% without source control and 14% with source control. Antibiotic studies also depict varying mortality rates (0–17%), although most of the studies report

mortality rates of less than 5%. Moreover, the success rates in clinical trials vary (80–100%), with the lowest success seen in cases of enterococci infection and post-operative peritonitis. These low success rates, however, are only detectable in subgroup analysis.

The choice of antibiotic regimens is very large due to reasons of study design, as mentioned earlier. The studies discussed earlier, comparing two different treatment regimens, are well characterized by a low Acute Physiology and Chronic Health Evaluation (APACHE) II score (ie, <10) and a high rate of peritonitis due to perforation of the appendix (24–60%). Such studies do not clarify the issue of whether to treat enteroccocci; however, there is no doubt that if cultured they would indicate that a patient has a significantly higher risk of infectious complications. This was found to be the case in one observational study, which looked at all cases of patients with peritonitis. This study by Wacha et al. (1999) showed a significant difference in APACHE II scores of the two collectives – one with enterococci and the other without enterococci (13.4 vs 10.0, respectively). The infection rates were also significantly different (63% vs 43%, respectively) with a p-value <0.05. Nonetheless, no significant difference in mortality was found (22% vs 15%). Another study by Wacha et al. (1999) showed identical mortality rates and a significant reduction in post-operative bacterial complications when enterococci were treated by administering adequate antibiotic treatment.

By contrast, a study by Röhrborn et al. (2000) found that there was no difference in outcome whether enterococci were treated or not. This was a prospective randomized study on intra-abdominal infection comparing antibiotic coverage with no antibiotic coverage of enterococci (penicillin-based vs cephalosporin-based); no difference between the treatment results was found. However, low-risk patients (APACHE II scores 9–10) and a low number of patients with enterococci were included in the study. Studies carried out by Solomkin et al. (1996) and Teppler et al. (2002) did not show any difference in the success rates whether enterococci were treated or not; however, success rates were lowest when compared with average rates or other collective studies.

Broad-spectrum antibiotic coverage seems to be the best choice in the treatment of intra-abdominal infection. Higher failure rates using limited-spectrum antibiotics should be expected, although Christou et al. (1996) found no difference in the failure rate between treatment groups comparing cefoxitin and imipenem, despite intra-operative cultures showing higher resistance rates against cefoxitin than against imipenem.

Empiric antibiotic treatment

Distinguishing between infectious processes and inflammatory processes is an important determinant; unlike inflammatory diseases, infectious diseases require treatment with antibiotics. Bowel injuries that are repaired within 12 hours and other intra-operative enteric contamination only require peri-operative antibiotic therapy for less than 24 hours. In addition, acute proximal gastro-intestinal perforations (eg, from the stomach, duodenum, and jejunum) require only 24 hours of prophylactic treatment. Acute cholecystitis and pancreatitis are inflammatory diseases and do not require antibiotic therapy unless the patient suffers a complication. Complicated disease processes, such as necrotizing pancreatitis, perforated appendicitis or diverticulitis, and infectious colitis, require timely and appropriate antibiotic coverage.

When should empiric antibiotic therapy be administered?

Once intra-abdominal infection is suspected, it is appropriate to start antibiotic therapy, even before an exact diagnosis is established or culture results are available. The goals of antibiotic therapy for intra-abdominal infection, in addition to source control, are to:

• eliminate infecting organisms;
• decrease the likelihood of recurrence; and
• shorten the time to resolution of signs and symptoms of infection.

Antibiotic therapy should begin after fluid resuscitation has been initiated, so that adequate visceral perfusion can be restored and better drug distribution is possible.

Choosing an empiric antibiotic regimen

For patients with mild-to-moderate community-acquired infections, antibiotics directed toward the likely organism based on the source of disease are the most effective. The stomach, duodenum, biliary tract and proximal small bowel are populated with gram-positive and gram-negative aerobic and facultative anaerobic organisms. The distal small bowel is a source of gram-negative aerobic and facultative anaerobic organisms, while the colon is the source of facultative and obligate anaerobic organisms, the most common being E. coli. Knowledge of the source of infection as well as the likely organism will guide antibiotic therapy toward these organisms. An antibiotic regimen should cover aerobic and anaerobic enteric flora. Single agents and combination therapy are both recommended because no regimen has been shown to be superior.

The severity of the infection will also determine the choice of antibiotic (*see* Figure 4.2). Antibiotic regimens for high-risk patients (those patients with APACHE II scores >10) are more or less based primarily on expert opinion and by taking into account the results from subgroups in large clinical trials. An important consideration is selecting antibiotic regimens that allow completion of therapy with oral forms of the drug, thereby allowing those patients with mild disease to complete a therapeutic course as an outpatient once an oral diet is tolerated (see 'Parenteral vs enteral administration' on page 62).

Despite the lack of evidence-based trials in all categories of intra-abdominal infections and the fact that trials often exclude severe cases, there are a number of agents that can be recommended for treatment and these are outlined in more detail in Appendix 1.

Recommended agents for the treatment of adults with community-acquired complicated intra-abdominal infections		
Regimen	Agents recommended for mild-to-moderate[†] infections	Agents recommended for high-risk or -severity[‡] infections
Single agent	Cefoxitin, ertapenem, moxifloxacin, tigecycline, and ticarcillin-clavulanic acid	Imipenem-cilastatin, meropenem, doripenem, and piperacillin-tazobactam
Combination	Cefazolin, cefuroxime, ceftriaxone, cefotaxime, ciprofloxacin, or levofloxacin, each in combination with metronidazole[*]	Cefepime, ceftazidime, ciprofloxacin, or levofloxacin, each in combination with metronidazole[*]

Figure 4.2 **Recommended agents for the treatment of adults with community-acquired complicated intra-abdominal infections.** [†]eg, perforated or abscessed appendicitis and other infections of mild-to-moderate severity; [‡]eg, severe physiologic disturbance, advanced age, or immunocompromised state. [*]Local population susceptibility profiles and, if available, isolate susceptibilty should be reviewed before use as there have been reports of an increased resistance of *Escherichia coli* to fluoroquinolones. Data from the Surgical Infection Society and the Infectious Diseases Society of America Guidelines. Diagnosis and Management of Complicated Intra-abdominal Infection in Adults and Children. Clin Infect Dis 2010; 50:133–64.

Therapeutic antimicrobial treatment

There are convincing data that the absence or inadequate use of empiric and definitive antibiotic therapy increases both treatment failure rates and mortality. By contrast, unnecessary or needlessly broad therapy is associated with bacterial resistance. The ideal goal is therefore to establish broad antibiotic coverage that is initially based on the likely pathogen for the disease process and the patient's specific comorbidities. The patient's response to therapy and the culture results will in turn enable antibiotic therapy to be better tailored to the specific needs of the patient.

Tailoring therapy

In community-acquired infections, the encountered flora is routinely susceptible to the recommended regimens. However, patients will frequently fail to improve or suffer a recurrence of the infection. In such circumstances it is important to follow and track any cultures obtained at the outset of therapy. Once culture results are available and antibiotic susceptibilities are known, therapy can be tailored to the specific organisms that are present. De-escalation of broad-spectrum antibiotic therapy may help to curb the rapid advance of bacterial resistance. Cultures should be obtained from the blood and any intra-abdominal fluid collections that have been drained, with the latter providing the greatest therapeutic guidance.

Duration of therapy

Antibiotic therapy for established infections should be continued until there is resolution of the clinical signs of infection, such as normalization of temperature and leukocyte count, and a return of gastrointestinal function. For patients who have persistent or recurrent clinical evidence of intra-abdominal infection following 5–7 days of therapy, appropriate diagnostic investigation should be undertaken. Adequate source control is essential and every effort to confirm drainage of intra-abdominal fluid should be taken, either with CT or abdominal ultrasound. If the patient has persistent clinical symptoms and signs but shows no evidence of a new or enduring infection, then antibiotic therapy can be terminated.

The duration of treatment in the comparative antibiotic studies discussed above ranged from 3 to 14 days. In contrast to these studies, clinical observation and some retrospective studies support the theory that the degree of antibiotic contamination is significantly associated with complications of post-operative infection and that a longer course of antibiotics was not associated with lower complications of infection. It is clear from antibiotic studies dealing with prophylaxis that a short contamination during operation or after trauma does not afford a prolongation of antibiotic administration for more than 24 hours. There is reasonable evidence that for some types of intra-abdominal infections, and where resection is possible, a short course of treatment can be advised. The antibiotics were recommended for a shorter time period of 3 days in acute appendicitis with perforation, gastroduodenal perforation, and sigma diverticulitis.

For penetrating abdominal trauma lasting 1–5 days regardless of the contamination and degree of injury, a 24-hour duration of antibiotics is sufficient. To shorten the duration of antibiotic therapy in intra-abdominal infections seems logical considering the following aspects:

• Studies from the pre-antibiotic era showed comparably good results.
• In the early stages of gastric perforation, antibiotics are not necessary.
• In ulcer perforation with a history of 12–24 hours, low numbers of anaerobic and aerobic gram-positive bacteria are treated easily by a short course of antibiotics.
• Bacterial numbers $<10^4$/mL are easily reduced by an intact immune defense alone.

In perforated appendicitis with diffuse peritonitis, selecting the right agent can shorten antibiotic therapy. Primary closure is standard in all practices of modern laparascopic appendectomy. In perforated appendicitis, mortality is rare; without antibiotics the mortality rate is 20–30%, and with certain antibiotic agents (eg, chloramphenicol, tetracyclines and sulfonamides), death can occur in 5–10% of cases, but these rates are continually being reduced with the introduction of better antibiotic agents and combination regimens using aminoglycoside, plus agents effective against anaerobes, resulting in mortality rates of 0–2%. Depending on the choice of agent and its spectrum of activity, antibiotics can reduce wound infection and abscess formation; for example, the intraperitoneal application of aminoglycoside as a single agent may reduce mortality but result in a high rate of wound infections and abscess formation (10–50%), which can only be reduced by administering aminoglycosan intravenously or as part of a combination therapy.

Similar observations can be made concerning stone obstruction in the biliary tract: a 3-day regimen of antibiotics is enough in cases where there is adequate drainage by endoscopic retrograde cholangiopancreaticography (ERCP). Van Lent (2002) reported that a short-duration (3-day course) of antibiotics was sufficient when adequate drainage was achieved and fever had abated. However, these recommendations do not apply to established long-term intra-abdominal infections.

How long should we treat severe infections (eg, with/without source control), post-operative infections, hospital-acquired infection, and so forth? Published studies support the trend to shorten the duration of antibiotic treatment, which was originally established at more than 10 days. In 1985, Stone reported that a patient was unlikely to experience recurrent sepsis when discontinuing antibiotic therapy if the following parameters were present:

• fever <38°C;
• a leukocyte count of 10,000/mL; and
• total granulocytes <60%.

However, even when these parameters are considered, a prefixed shorter course of antibiotics seems to show better results, as highlighted in a recent retrospective study by Hedrick et al. (2006), which supported the benefits of a shorter course of antibiotics. In this study, the authors evaluated the data from 5561 treated infections and, for all infections, whether analyzed by absolute duration, time from resolution of leukocytosis (>11,000/mL) or fever (>38°C), the shorter course of antibiotic treatment of less than 12 days was associated with the lowest recurrence rates (14–23%). Individual analysis of intra-abdominal infections and pneumonia yielded similar results. Furthermore, additional clinical parameters besides fever and leukocytes were also demonstrated to be of some value in deciding to stop antibiotic therapy. To find the appropriate duration for the individual patient with an intra-abdominal infection, basic information derived from empirical studies are invaluable.

Wacha and Helm (1982) studied the efficacy of different antibiotics in the common bile duct in a clinical setting; tetracycline and aminoglycoside administered parenterally were found to have no impact on reducing organisms in bile. In cases of successful surgical decompression, adequate antibiotic therapy resulted in reduction and elimination of organisms in bile within 24 hours. In cases of stone obstruction, there was no visible change of bacterial growth, even when the antibiotic agent chosen was the most appropriate for treatment. One of the earliest studies to compare short- and long-term courses of antibiotic administration following experimental peritonitis was published in 1977; the experiments in this study demonstrated higher survival rates and smaller abscess size with administration of clindamycin and tobramycin over 2 days when compared with a regimen lasting 2–7 days.

Further experimental data studying the duration of therapy are lacking. It would be interesting to study the timely correlation between the duration of bacterial infection and onset of therapy, as well as the optimum length of therapy. It is the experience of the authors that a much shorter treatment time is sufficient in the average case where the patient has intact organ function and has received adequate surgical intervention and intensive care measures. We need to change our strategy of simply killing bacteria to one where we think much more about restricting prescriptions and adopting shorter courses of antibiotic regimens. Antibiosis should not be our aim, but instead a form of symbiosis; antibiotic treatment should not cause indefinable collateral damage to the patient.

Parenteral vs enteral administration

The concentrations of parenterally administered antibiotics in the peritoneal fluid exceeds the MIC of most organisms found in peritonitis. Even when antibiotics are administered intraperitoneally, neither higher doses of the antibiotic nor improved effectiveness are required. Discussions concerning extended lavage with or without antibiotics should be confined to the past. Extended lavage without antibiotics failed to significantly reduce the mesothelial microbial population, whereas antimicrobial lavage produced an immediate decrease in mesothelial microbial recovery. These results, however, were transitory; the microbial population 24 hours post-lavage remained the same as, or exceeded, the pre-lavage levels.

In daily practice, adequate serum, tissue, and antibiotic levels over the MIC can be achieved securely by parenteral administration of the antibiotics. In rare instances, oral intake may be a possibility, but only if the gastrointestinal tract is functioning properly. Agents with comparably good bioavailability (ie, equally high levels whether administered orally or parentally) should be selected (eg, quinolones, metronidazole); for example, bioavailability with ciprofloxacin was shown when given in a 750 mg dose twice-daily by enteral feeding through a tube and 400 mg twice-daily administered intravenously. One clinical trial also showed the same results with 500 mg metronidazole, taken orally, when compared to a combination of ceftizoxime with penicillin and chloramphenicol in perforated appendicitis. In cases of complicated intra-abdominal infection, a switch from intravenous to oral treatment is possible after 4 or 5 days, if the patient is able to tolerate oral feedings, with a combination of ciprofloxacin/metronidazole, which provided similar results to ceftriaxone/metronidazole, and imipenem/cilastin. High doses can only be achieved parenterally, and quinolones and aminoglycosides should therefore be administered once daily.

It can be difficult to determine the right dose of a given antibiotic for each patient. Patients with severe peritonitis develop substantial fluid sequestration. The inflammatory mediators released in the systemic inflammatory response syndrome result in widespread capillary leak syndrome and inadequate tissue perfusion. In cases of severe sepsis, the dose of aminoglycosides should be increased to six times the standard dose (eg, a 5 mg/kg dose should be increased to 30 mg/kg).

Taking into consideration the high-colony counts of organisms and agents at the beginning of therapy and the immunomodulating effect of the surgeon by entering the abdomen, it is worth giving the first dose intra-operatively after confirming the diagnosis and beginning surgical source-control management. This must be considered in the emergency care setting, where the patient has only had a short disease history, for example in cases with a short history of peritonitis and immediate operation under optimal conditions. The use of combination therapy to overcome potentially resistant organisms is also a possibility.

Antibiotic treatment and outcome

Generally, inadequate antibiotic treatment leads to a poorer outcome (which seems to be true in the case of ventilator-associated pneumonia) and affects mortality. By contrast, in the case of intra-abdominal infection, an inappropriate antibiotic regimen has only a modest impact on outcome and does not affect mortality. Surgical treatment reduces the bacterial load and ensures source control in 14–47% of cases. There are only a few studies that have evaluated the effects, based on culture results, of a change of antibiotic agent on outcome. Similarly, few reports have studied the relationship between the adequacy of initial empirically based antibiotic therapy and outcome. In the case of peritonitis, these studies showed no significant influence on post-operative outcome (eg, post-operative complications).

In one retrospective study, Sotto et al. (2002) showed that there was no difference in the mortality rate between patients whose post-operative treatment was changed following results from intra-operative peritoneal cultures and patients receiving inappropriate antibiotic treatment.

In another study, Barie et al. (2005) reported a 94% rate of 'appropriate' antibiotic therapy using a scheduled monthly antibiotic cycle. The mortality rate among these severely ill patients in an intensive care unit setting was 31% and this rate was not shown to be influenced by inappropriate antibiotic therapy. The initial administration of antibiotics does not appear to be crucial for survival and neither is the site of infection nor any specific pathogen. The antibiotics used included vancomycin (30%), piperacillin/tazobactam (18%), carpenem (16%), quinolone (14%), and cefipime (7%), to name but a few. Barie et al. define clinical appropriateness as a higher cure rate (measured using various clinical parameters) than expected in the clinical setting given the resistance patterns of the organisms presumed to be responsible for the infection. The percentage of clinically appropriate antibiotic therapy was 5–10% higher than microbiological appropriateness, especially in treatment with cefipime and vancomycin, and the mortality attributed to these two antibiotics was significantly higher ($p<0.01$).

Montravers et al. (1996) evaluated cases of post-operative peritonitis, and reported that inadequate empirical treatment was associated with a significantly poorer outcome (45% mortality) compared with adequate empirical therapy (16% mortality); according to culture results, a change in antibiotic regimen had no effect on outcome.

In a more recently published study by Krobot et al. (2004), inappropriate therapy was significantly associated with additional antibiotic therapy, unscheduled repeated operations or mortality of any cause. Data from 20 clinics across Germany comprising 425 patients with community-acquired intra-abdominal infection with adequate source control, were analyzed after adjusting for gender, age, and comorbidity. Ampicillin/sulbactam, amoxicillin/clavulanate, imipenem, piperacillin/tazobactam and cefotaxim were used as monotherapy. Combination therapy with metronidazole was documented with cefotaxim, cefuroxime, cefazolin, piperacillin/tazobactam, mezlocillin, amoxicillin/clavulanate, and ceftriaxon. The conclusions drawn from these experiments are that neither the spectrum of the antibiotic agent being used nor the resistance pattern alone influence outcome. Clearly, adequate therapy for treating intra-abdominal infections is a far more complex decision. The choice of antibiotic agent is an individual decision, which takes into account the severity of the patient, the cause of the disease, surgical treatment options, and geographic variations in resistance patterns. There are some principles to guide choosing the most appropriate antibiotic agent but the decision is largely based on experience and empirical evidence.

Special considerations
Identifying high-risk patients

Patients predicted to have a worse than usual outcome from intra-abdominal infection warrant a treatment regimen with broad-spectrum antimicrobial activity. Patients deserving special consideration are those with higher APACHE II scores (ie, >10), poor nutrition, significant cardiovascular disease, inadequate source control, and immunosuppression due to transplantation or chronic illness.

Several scoring systems are used to assess the risk of mortality from intra-abdominal infections. Two of the most widely used scoring systems are the Mannheim Peritonitis Index (MPI) (*see* Figure 4.3) and the APACHE II (*see* Figure 4.4), both of which have been evaluated in numerous clinical studies. The MPI counts independent risk factors by statistical analysis, and the APACHE II evaluates risk factors by expert opinion and statistical analysis. Patients with high score values (eg, APACHE II score >10, MPI >15) are at an increased risk of developing tertiary peritonitis (*see* Figure 1.3). Recurrent infections characterized by an overgrowth of *Candida* spp. and multiresistant organisms are the most difficult to treat infectious complications and prophylaxis must include early, adequate and optimal surgical and antibiotic therapy.

The Mannheim Peritonitis Index	
Risk factor	Weighting if present
Age >50 years	5
Female sex	5
Organ failure*	7
Malignancy	4
Pre-operative duration of peritonitis >24 h	4
Origin of sepsis not colonic	4
Diffuse generalized peritonitis	6
Exudate	
Clear	0
Cloudy, purulent	6
Fecal	12

*Definitions of organ failure include:
- kidney: creatinine level ≥177 μmol/l, urea level ≥167 mmol/l, oliguria <20 ml/h
- lung: partial pressure of oxygen <50 mmHg, partial pressure of carbon dioxide >50 mmHg
- hypodynamic or hyperdynamic shock
- intestinal obstruction: paralysis ≥24 h or complete mechanical ileus

Figure 4.3 The Mannheim Peritonitis Index. Reproduced with permission from Billing A, Fröhlich D, The Peritonitis Study Group. Prediction of outcome using the Mannheim peritonitis index in 2003 patients. Br J Surg 1994; 81:209–13.

Healthcare-associated infections

Infections occurring after elective or emergent surgery or in patients continually hospitalized due to chronic infection convey a more resistant flora than is routinely encountered in the community. Antibiotic therapy for such infections should be guided by knowledge of the nosocomial flora seen in each hospital and microbial susceptibilities. Often, this may require the use of multi-drug regimens.

APACHE II severity of disease classification system

Physiological parameter	High abnormal range				0	Low abnormal range				Points
	+4	+3	+2	+1		+1	+2	+3	+4	
Temperature – rectal (°C)	≥41	39–40.9		38.5–38.9	36–38.4	34–35.9	32–33.9	30–31.9	≤29.9	
Mean arterial pressure (mmHg)	≥160	130–159	110–129		70–109		50–69		≤49	
Heart rate (ventricular response)	≥180	140–179	110–139		70–109		55–69	40–54	≤39	
Respiratory rate (non-ventilated or ventilated)	≥50	35–49		25–34	12–24	10–11	6–9		≤5	
Oxygenation: A–aDO$_2$ or PaO$_2$ (mmHg) a. FiO$_2$ ≥0.5 record A–aDO$_2$ b. FiO$_2$ <0.5 record only PaO$_2$	≥500	350–499	200–349		<200 / PO$_2$ >70	PO$_2$ 61–70		PO$_2$ 55–60	PO$_2$ <55	
Arterial pH	≥7.7	7.6–7.69		7.5–7.59	7.33–7.49		7.25–7.32	7.15–7.24	<7.15	
Serum HCO$_3$ (venous mMol/L) (not preferred, but use if no ABGs)	≥52	41–51.9		32–40.9	22–31.9		18–21.9	15–17.9	<15	
Serum sodium (mMol/L)	≥180	160–179	155–159	150–154	130–149		120–129	111–119	≤110	
Serum potassium (mMol/L)	≥7	6–6.9		5.5–5.9	3.5–5.4	3–3.4	2.5–2.9		<2.5	
Serum creatinine (mg/100ml) (double point score for acute renal failure)	≥3.5	2–3.4	1.5–1.9		0.6–1.4		<0.6			
Hematocrit (%)	≥60		50–59.9	46–49.9	30–45.9		20–29.9		<20	
White blood count (total/mm³) (in 1000s)	≥40		20–39.9	15–19.9	3–14.9		1–2.9		<1	

Glasgow Coma Score (GCS):
Score = 15 minus actual GCS

A – Total Acute Physiology Score = (sum of above points)	A
B – Age points (years) Assign points to age as follows: <44=0, 45–54=2, 55–64=3, 65–74=5, ≥75=6	B
C – Chronic health points If the patient has a history of severe organ system insufficiency* or is immunocompromised* assign points as follows: 5 points for non-operative or emergency postoperative patients 2 points for elective postoperative patients	C

*Definitions: organ insufficiency or immunocompromised state must have been evident prior to this hospital admission and conform to the following criteria:
- Liver – biopsy proven cirrhosis and documented portal hypertension; episodes of past upper GI bleeding attributed to portal hypertension; or prior episodes of hepatic failure/encephalopathy/coma.
- Cardiovascular – New York Heart Association Class IV.
- Respiratory – Chronic restrictive, obstructive, or vascular disease resulting in severe exercise restriction (ie, unable to climb stairs or perform household duties; or documented chronic hypoxia, hypercapnia, secondary polycythemia, severe pulmonary hypertension (>40 mmHg), or respirator dependency.
- Renal – receiving chronic dialysis.
- Immunocompromised – the patient has received therapy that suppresses resistance to infection (eg, immunosuppression, chemotherapy, radiation, long-term or recent high-dose steroids, or has a disease that is sufficiently advanced to suppress resistance to infection, eg, leukemia, lymphoma, AIDS).

Total APACHE II score =	A+B+C

Figure 4.4 APACHE II severity of disease classification system. A–aDO$_2$, alveolar-arterial oxygen tension difference, ABGs, arterial blood gas tests ; APACHE, Acute Physiology and Chronic Health Evaluation; FiO$_2$, fraction of inspired oxygen; GI, gastrointestinal; HCO$_3$, hydrogen carbonate; PO$_2$, partial pressure of oxygen in arterial blood. APACHE II: a severity of disease classification. Crit Care Med 1985; 13: 818–29. Reproduced with permission from Knaus et al.

Appendix

The table below outlines in detail antibiotic agents used for the treatment of intra-abdominal infections. It is important to note that not all antibiotics are available in all countries. Local resistance patterns must also be taken into consideration when choosing the most appropriate antibiotic agent.

Antibiotic agents for the treatment of intra-abdominal infections	
Carbapenems	
Imipenem/cilastatin	
Spectrum	Gram-positives, gram-negatives (including *Pseudomonas*), anaerobes
Pharmacokinetic parameters	
Protein binding	Imipenem 20%, cilastatin 40%
Volume of distribution	0.15–0.25 l/kg
Metabolism	Kidney: extensive
Excretion	Renal excretion: imipenem 50–70%, cilastatin 70–75%
Elimination half-life	1 h
Daily dose and interval	500 mg/6 h–1000 mg/8 h
Meropenem	
Spectrum	Gram-positives, gram-negatives (incl. *Pseudomonas*), anaerobes
Pharmacokinetic parameters	
Protein binding	2%
Volume of distribution	0.15–0.3 l/kg
Metabolism	Extrarenal: 20–25%
Excretion	Renal excretion: 60–80%
Elimination half-life	1 h
Daily dose and interval	1 g/8 h

Appendix 1 Antibiotic agents for the treatment of intra-abdominal infections. Continued on next page.

Ertapenem

Spectrum	Gram-positives, gram-negatives (excl. *Pseudomonas*), anaerobes
Pharmacokinetic parameters	
Protein binding	85–95 %
Volume of distribution	0.1 l/kg
Metabolism	Kidney: moderate
Excretion	Renal excretion: >80%; bile: approximately 10%
Elimination half-life	4 h
Daily dose and interval	1 g/24 h

Aminopenicillins/β-lactamase inhibitors

Ampicillin/sulbactam

Spectrum	Gram-positives (incl. *Enterococcus* spp., MSSA/MSSE), gram-negatives, anaerobes. Can be hydrolysed by β-lactamases eg, *Staphylococcus*, *Escherichia coli*, *Proteus* spp. and *Bacteroides* spp., and therefore should be used in fixed combinations with a β-lactamase inhibitor
Pharmacokinetic parameters	
Protein binding	Ampicillin 17–28%, sulbactam 38%
Volume of distribution	Ampicillin 0.2–0.3 l/kg, sulbactam 0.2–0.3 l/kg
Metabolism	Liver: ampicillin 10–20 %, sulbactam 38%
Excretion	Renal excretion: ampicillin and sulbactam 75–85%, bile: 2.8% of ampicillin, 1% of sulbactam
Elimination half-life	Ampicillin 0.7–1.2 h, sulbactam 0.5–1 h
Daily dose and interval	1.5–3 g/8 h

Amoxicillin/clavulanic acid

Spectrum	Gram-positives (incl. *Enterococcus* spp., MSSA/MSSE), gram-negatives, anaerobes. Can be hydrolysed by β-lactamases eg, *Staphylococcus*, *Escherichia coli*, *Proteus* spp. and *Bacteroides* spp., and therefore should be used in fixed combinations with a β-lactamase inhibitor

Appendix 1 (continued) Antibiotic agents for the treatment of intra-abdominal infections.
MSSA, methicillin-sensitive *Staphylococcus aureus*; MSSE, methicillin-sensitive *Staphylococcus epidermidis*. Continued on next page.

Pharmacokinetic parameters

Protein binding	Amoxicillin 18 %, clavulanic acid 25%
Volume of distribution	Amoxicillin 0.2–0.3 l/kg; clavulanic acid 0.3 l/kg
Metabolism	Liver: extensively
Excretion	Renal excretion: amoxicillin 50–70%, clavulanic acid 25–40%
Elimination half-life	Amoxicillin 1 h, clavulanic acid 1–1.5 h
Daily dose and interval	1.2–2.2 g/8 h

Ticarcillin/clavulanic acid

Spectrum	Gram-positives (incl. *Enterococcus* spp., MSSA/MSSE), gram-negatives, anaerobes. Can be hydrolysed by β-lactamases eg, *Staphylococcus*, *Escherichia coli*, *Proteus* spp. and *Bacteroides* spp., and therefore should be used in fixed combinations with a β-lactamase inhibitor

Pharmacokinetic parameters

Protein binding	Ticarcillin 45%, clavulanic acid 25%
Volume of distribution	Ticarcillin 1.5 l/kg, clavulanic acid 0.3 l/kg
Metabolism	Liver: extensive
Excretion	Renal excretion: ticarcillin 60–77%, clavulanic acid 35–45%
Elimination half-life	Ticarcillin 1 h, clavulanic acid 1–1.5 h
Daily dose and interval	3.1 g/6 h

Acylaminopenicillins/β-lactamase inhibitors

Piperacillin/tazobactam

Spectrum	Gram-negatives (incl. *Pseudomonas*) gram-positives (incl. *Enterococcus* spp., MSSA/MSSE), anaerobes. Can be hydrolysed by β-lactamases eg, *Staphylococcus*, *Escherichia coli*, *Proteus* spp. and *Bacteroides* spp., and therefore should be used combined with sulbactam or in fixed combinations with the β-lactamase inhibitor tazobactam

Appendix 1 (continued) Antibiotic agents for the treatment of intra-abdominal infections.
MSSA, methicillin-sensitive *Staphylococcus aureus*; MSSE, methicillin-sensitive *Staphylococcus epidermidis*. Continued on next page.

Pharmacokinetic parameters

Protein binding	Piperacillin 30%, tazobactam 30%
Volume of distribution	0.2–0.3 l/kg
Metabolism	Liver: piperacillin small amount, tazobactam extensively
Excretion	Renal excretion: piperacillin 80%, bile: 10–20%
Elimination half-life	1 h
Daily dose and interval	4.5 g/6 h

Mezlocillin + sulbactam

Spectrum	Gram-negatives, gram-positives (incl. *Enterococcus* spp., MSSA/MSSE), anaerobes. Can be hydrolysed by β-lactamases eg, *Staphylococcus*, *Escherichia coli*, *Proteus* spp. and *Bacteroides* spp., and therefore should be used in combination with sulbactam

Pharmacokinetic parameters

Protein binding	Mezlocillin 30–40%, sulbactam 40%
Volume of distribution	Mezlocillin 0.1–0.2 l/kg, sulbactam 0.2–0.3 l/kg
Metabolism	Mezlocillin 50%, sulbactam 40 %
Excretion	Renal excretion: mezlocillin 60–70%, bile: sulbactam 25%
Elimination half-life	Mezlocillin 1 h, sulbactam 1 h
Daily dose and interval	2 (4) + 0.5 g/8 h maximal dose in therapy for intra-abdominal infection preferable

Cephalosporins (second-generation)

Cefuroxime

Spectrum	Gram positives (excl. *Enterococcus* spp., MRSA/ MRSE), gram-negatives

Pharmacokinetic parameters

Protein binding	30%
Volume of distribution	0.2–0.3 l/kg
Metabolism	Small amount
Excretion	Renal excretion: 90%
Elimination half-life	1–1.5 h
Daily dose and interval	1.5 g/8 h

Appendix 1 (continued) Antibiotic agents for the treatment of intra-abdominal infections. MRSA, methicillin-resistant *Staphylococcus aureus*; MRSE, methicillin-resistant *Staphylococcus epidermidis*; MSSA, methicillin-sensitive *Staphylococcus aureus*; MSSE, methicillin-sensitive *Staphylococcus epidermidis*. Continued on next page.

Cephalosporins (third-generation)

Ceftriaxone

Spectrum	Gram-negatives, gram-positives (excl. *Enterococcus* spp., MRSA/MRSE; poor activity against MSSA, MSSE)
Pharmacokinetic parameters	
Protein binding	85–95%
Volume of distribution	0.12–0.18 l/kg
Metabolism	Apparently metabolized in intestine after biliary excretion
Excretion	Renal excretion: 35–65 %, bile: 35–45%
Elimination half-life	5.8–8.7 h
Daily dose and interval	1–2 (4) g/24 h

Cefotaxime

Spectrum	Gram-negatives, gram-positives (excl. *Enterococcus* spp., MRSA/MRSE; poor activity against MSSA, MSSE)
Pharmacokinetic parameters	
Protein binding	30–40%
Volume of distribution	0.4 l/kg
Metabolism	Liver: about 50%
Excretion	Renal excretion: 50–85%
Elimination half-life	0.8–1.4 h
Daily dose and interval	1–2 g/8 h

Ceftazidime

Spectrum	Gram-negatives (incl. *Pseudomonas*), gram-positives (excl. *Enterococcus* spp., MRSA/MRSE poor activity against MSSA, MSSE)
Pharmacokinetic parameters	
Protein binding	5–17%
Volume of distribution	0.25–0.4 l/kg
Metabolism	Not metabolized
Excretion	Renal excretion: 90–96%
Elimination half-life	1.6–2 h
Daily dose and interval	2 g/8h

Appendix 1 (continued) Antibiotic agents for the treatment of intra-abdominal infections. MRSA, methicillin-resistant *Staphylococcus aureus*; MRSE, methicillin-resistant *Staphylococcus epidermidis*; MSSA, methicillin-sensitive *Staphylococcus aureus*; MSSE, methicillin-sensitive *Staphylococcus epidermidis*. Continued on next page.

Cephalosporins (fourth-generation)

Cefepime

Spectrum	Gram-negatives (incl. *Pseudomonas*), gram-positives (excl. *Enterococcus* spp., MRSA/MRSE)
Pharmacokinetic parameters	
Protein binding	16–20%
Volume of distribution	0.2–0.3 l/kg
Metabolism	Liver: partially
Excretion	Renal excretion: 70–99%
Elimination half-life	4 h
Daily dose and interval	2 g/12 h

Fluoroquinolones

Ciprofloxacin

Spectrum	Gram-negatives (incl. *Pseudomonas*), atypical bacteria
Pharmacokinetic parameters	
Protein binding	20–40%
Volume of distribution	1.2–2.7 l/kg
Metabolism	Liver: significant
Excretion	Renal excretion: 30–57%, feces: 20–35%, bile: small amount
Elimination half-life	3–6 h
Daily dose and interval	400 mg every 8–12 h in combination with metronidazole

Ofloxacin

Spectrum	Gram-negatives, atypical bacteria
Pharmacokinetic parameters	
Protein binding	20–32%
Volume of distribution	1.5–2 l/kg
Metabolism	Liver, minimal
Excretion	Renal excretion: 72–98.5%; feces: 4–8%
Elimination half-life	5–7.5 h
Daily dose and interval	400 mg/24 h

Appendix 1 (continued) Antibiotic agents for the treatment of intra-abdominal infections.
MRSA, methicillin-resistant *Staphylococcus aureus*; MRSE, methicillin-resistant *Staphylococcus epidermidis*; Continued on next page.

Moxifloxacin

Spectrum	Gram-positives, gram-negatives (excl. *Pseudomonas*), atypical bacteria, anaerobes
Pharmacokinetic parameters	
Protein binding	30–50 %
Volume of distribution	1.7–2.7 l/kg
Metabolism	Liver 52 %
Excretion	Renal excretion: 38% (22% unchanged), feces: 61% (26% unchanged)
Elimination half-life	10–14 h
Daily dose and interval	400 mg/24 h

Glycylcycline

Tigecycline

Spectrum	Gram-positives (incl. MRSA, MRSE, VRE), gram-negatives (excl. *Pseudomonas*, *Proteus* spp.), anaerobes
Pharmacokinetic parameters	
Protein binding	70–90%
Volume of distribution	7–9 l/kg
Metabolism	Not extensively metabolized
Excretion	Renal excretion: 33%, bile: 59%
Elimination half-life	42 h
Daily dose and interval	Initial 100 mg, followed by 50 mg/12 h

Nitroimidazole

Metronidazole

Spectrum	Anaerobes
Pharmacokinetic parameters	
Protein binding	10–20%
Volume of distribution	0.5 l/kg
Metabolism	Liver: extensive
Excretion	Renal excretion: 80 %
Elimination half-life	8 h
Daily dose and interval	In combination with a β-lactam antibiotic 0.5 g/8 h

Appendix 1 (continued) Antibiotic agents for the treatment of intra-abdominal infections.
MRSA, methicillin-resistant *Staphylococcus aureus*; MRSE, methicillin-resistant *Staphylococcus epidermidis*; VRE, vancomycin-resistant *Enterococci*. Continued on next page.

Aminoglycosides	
Gentamicin	
Spectrum	Gram-negatives, less active against gram-positives
Pharmacokinetic parameters	
Protein binding	<10%
Volume of distribution	0.25 l/kg
Metabolism	Not metabolized
Excretion	Renal excretion: >90%
Elimination half-life	2 h
Daily dose and interval	5–7 mg/kg preferable once daily dosing; drug monitoring after 3–5 days necessary; †trough level: <1 mg/l; *peak level: 20–25 mg/l
Tobramycin	
Spectrum	Gram-negatives (best activity against *Pseudomonas aeruginosa* among aminoglycosides), less active against gram-positives
Pharmacokinetic parameters	
Protein binding	<10%
Volume of distribution	0.25 l/kg
Metabolism	Not metabolized
Excretion	Renal excretion: >90%
Elimination half-life	2 h
Daily dose and interval	5–7 mg/kg preferable once daily dosing, drug monitoring after 3–5 days necessary; †trough level: <1 mg/l; *peak level: 20–25 mg/l
Amikacin	
Spectrum	Gram-negatives (good activity against *Pseudomonas aeruginosa*), less active against gram-positives
Pharmacokinetic parameters	
Protein binding	<10%
Volume of distribution	0.25 l/kg
Metabolism	Not metabolized
Excretion	Renal excretion: >90%
Elimination half-life	2 h
Daily dose and interval	15–20 mg/kg preferable once daily dosing, drug monitoring after 3–5 days necessary; †trough level: <2(1) mg/l; *peak level: 55–60 mg/l

Appendix 1 (continued) Antibiotic agents for the treatment of intra-abdominal infections. †Trough level is the lowest level of a medicine that is present in the body and for any antibiotic administered periodically the trough level should be measured prior to the next dose to prevent overdosing. *Peak level is the highest level of the antibiotic agent medicine in the body.

Suggested reading

Alcocer F, Lopez E, Calva JJ et al. [Antibiotic therapy in secondary peritonitis: towards a definition of its optimal duration.] Rev Invest Clin 2001; 53:121–5.

Al-Nassir WN, Sethi AK, Nerandzic MM. Comparison of clinical and microbiological response to treatment of clostridium difficile–associated disease with metronidazole and vancomycin. Clin Infect Dis 2008; 47:56–62.

Alverdy JC, Aoys E, Moss GS. Total parenteral nutrition promotes bacterial translocation from the gut. Surgery 1988; 104:185–90.

Andaker L, Kling PA, Burman LG. Antibiotic consumption and faecal bacterial susceptibility in surgical in-patients. Acta Chir Scand 1987; 153:411–6.

Andaker L, Hojer H, Kihlstrom E et al. Stratified duration of prophylactic antimicrobial treatment in emergency abdominal surgery. Metronidazole-fosfomycin vs. metronidazole-gentamicin in 381 patients. Acta Chir Scand 1987; 153:185–92.

Bailey JA, Virgo KS, DiPiro JT et al. Aminoglycosides for intra-abdominal infection: equal to the challenge? Surg Infect (Larchmt) 2002; 3:315–35.

Banani SA, Talei A. Can oral metronidazole substitute parenteral drug therapy in acute appendicitis? A new policy in the management of simple or complicated appendicitis with localized peritonitis: a randomized controlled clinical trial. Am Surg 1999; 65:411–6.

Barie PS, Hydo LJ, Shou J et al. Influence of antibiotic therapy on mortality of critical surgical illness caused or complicated by infection. Surg Infect (Larchmt) 2005; 6:41–54.

Bartlett JG, Louie TJ, Gorbach SL et al. Therapeutic efficacy of 29 antimicrobial regimens in experimental intraabdominal sepsis. Rev Infect Dis 1981; 3:535–42.

Beger HG, Bittner R, Block S et al. Bacterial contamination of pancreatic necrosis. A prospective clinical study. Gastroenterology 1986; 91:433–8.

Berg DF, Bahadursingh AM, Kaminksi DL. Acute surgical emergencies in inflammatory bowel disease. Am J Surgery 2002; 184:45–51.

Billing A, Fröhlich D, The Peritonitis Study Group. Prediction of outcome using the Mannheim peritonitis index in 2003 patients. Peritonitis Study Group. Br J Surgery 1994; 81:209–13.

Boey J, Wong J. Perforated duodenal ulcers. World J Surg 1987; 11:319–24.

Branicki FJ, Coleman SY, Fok PJ et al. Bleeding peptic ulcer: a prospective evaluation of risk factors for rebleeding and mortality. World J Surg 1990; 14:262–9.

Bucher P, Mermillod B, Gervaz P et al. Mechanical bowel preparation for elective colorectal surgery: a meta-analysis. Arch Surg 2004; 139:1359–64.

Christou NV, Turgeon P, Wassef et al. Management of intra-abdominal infections. The case for intraoperative cultures and comprehensive broad-spectrum antibiotic coverage. The Canadian Intra-abdominal Infection Study Group. Arch Surg 1996; 131:1193–201.

Condon RE, Wittmann DH. The use of antibiotics in general surgery. Curr Probl Surg 1991; 28:801–949.

Cunningham R, Dial S. Is over-use of proton pump inhibitors fuelling the current epidemic of clostridium difficile-associated diarrhoea? J Hosp Infec 2008; 70:1–6.

Davis et al. Gastroenterology and hepatology: gallbladder and bile ducts. Edited by M Feldman, NF LaRusso. Philadelphia: Current Medicine LLC, 1997.

De Dombal FT. Diagnosis of acute abdominal pain. New York: Churchill Livingstone 1991.

De Marie S, VandenBergh MF, Buijk SL et al. Bioavailability of ciprofloxacin after multiple enteral and intravenous doses in ICU patients with severe gram-negative intra-abdominal infections. Intensive Care Med 1998; 24:343–6.

Demmel N, Muth G, Maag K et al. [Prognostic scores in peritonitis: the Mannheim Peritonitis Index or APACHE II?] Langenbecks Arch Chirg 1994; 379:347–52.

Desai DC, Brennan EJ Jr, Reilly JF et al. The utility of the Hartmann procedure. Am J Surg 1998; 175:152–4.

Ding LA, Li JS. Intestinal failure: pathophysiological elements and clinical diseases. World J Gastroenterol 2004; 10:930–3.

Edmiston, CE, Goheen, MP, Kornhall S et al. Fecal peritonitis: microbial adherence to serosal mesothelium and resistance to peritoneal lavage. World J Surg 1990; 14:176–83.

Eriksson S, Granström L. Randomized controlled trial of appendicectomy versus antibiotic therapy for acute appendicitis. Br J Surg 1995; 82:166–9.

Esposito C, Borzi P, Valla JS et al. Laparoscopic versus open appendectomy in children: a retrospective comparative study of 2,332 cases. World J Surg 2007; 31:750–5.

Fabian TC, Croce MA, Payne LW et al. Duration of antibiotic therapy for penetrating abdominal trauma: a prospective trial. Surgery 1992; 112:788–94.

Finegold et al. Intra-abdominal infections and abscesses. In: Atlas of infectious diseases: intra-abdominal infections, hepatitis, and gastroenteritis. Edited by G Mandell, B Lorber. Philadelphia: Current Medicine LLC, 1997.

Finegold SM, Wilson SE. In: Atlas of infectious diseases: intra-abdominal infections, hepatitis, and gastroenteritis. Edited by B Lorber. Current Medicine, Inc. 2000.

Flum DR, Morris A, Koepsell T et al. Has misdiagnosis of appendicitis decreased over time? A population-based analysis. JAMA 2001; 286:1748–53.

Fry DE. Preventive systemic antibiotics in colorectal surgery. Surg Infect (Larchmt) 2008; 9:547–52.

Garibaldi RA, Cushing D, Lerer T. Risk factors for postoperative infection. Am J Med 1991; 91:158S–163S.

Giger U, Michel JM, Vonlanthen R et al. Laparoscopic cholecystectomy in acute cholecystitis: indication, technique, risk and outcome. Langenbecks Arch Surg 2005; 390:373–80.

Gleisner AL, Argenta R, Pimentel M et al. Infective complications according to duration of antibiotic treatment in acute abdomen. Int J Infect Dis 2004; 8:155–62.

Gloor B, Müller CA, Worni M et al. Late mortality in patients with severe acute pancreatitis. Br J Surg 2001; 88:975–9.

Golub R, Siddiqi F, Pohl D et al. Role of antibiotics in acute pancreatitis: a meta-analysis. J Gastrointest Surg 1998; 2:496–503.

Graham et al. Atlas of infectious diseases: intra-abdominal infections, hepatitis, and gastroenteritis. Edited by G Mandell, B Lorber. Philadelphia: Current Medicine LLC, 1997.

Hau T, Ohmann C, Wolmershauser A et al. Planned relaparotomy vs. relaparotomy on demand in the treatment of intra-abdominal infections. The peritonitis study group of the surgical infection society-europe. Arch Surg 1995; 130:1193–6.

Hedrick TL, Evans HL, Smith RL et al. Can we define the ideal duration of therapy? Surg Infect (Larchmt) 2006; 7:419–32.

Hess W, Rohnen A, Cirenei A et al. Die Erkrankungen der Gallenwege und des Pankreas. Padua: Piccini Nueva Libera, 1985.

Hinchey EJ, Schaal PG, Richards GK. Treatment of perforated diverticular disease of the colon. Adv Surg 1978; 1012:85–109.

Holzheimer RG, Dralle H. Paradigm change in 30 years peritonitis treatment – a review on source control. Eur J Med Res 2001; 6:161–8.

Hunt JL. Generalized peritonitis. To irrigate or not to irrigate the abdominal cavity. Arch Surg 1982; 117:209–12.

Isenmann R, Beger HG. Bacterial infection of pancreatic necrosis: role of bacterial translocation, impact of antibiotic treatment. Pancreatology 2001; 1:79–89.

Itani KMF, Kim L. Mechanical bowel preparation or not for elective colorectal surgery. Surg Infect (Larchmt) 2008; 9: 563–5.

Kalfarentzos F, Kehagias J, Mead N et al. Enteral nutrition is superior to parenteral nutrition in severe acute pancreatitis: Results of a randomized prospective trial. Br J Surg 1997; 84:1665–9.

Kanwar S, Windsor AC, Welsh F et al. Lack of correlation between failure of gut barrier function and septic complications after major upper gastrointestinal surgery. Ann Surg 2000; 231:88–95.

Khan AL, Ah-See AK, Crofts TJ et al. Reversal of Hartmann's colostomy. J R Coll Surg Edinb 1994; 39:239–42.

Kirshtein B, Bayme M, Domchik S et al. Complicated appendicitis: laparoscopic or conventional Surgery? World J Surg 2007; 31:744–9.

Knaus WA, Draper EA, Wagner DR et al. APACHE II: a severity of disease classification system. Crit Care Med 1985; 13:818–29.

Knaus WA, Wagner DP, Draper EA et al. The APACHE III prognostic system. Risk prediction of hospital mortality for critically ill hospitalized adults. Chest 1991; 100:1619–36.

Kollef MH. Antibiotic management of ventilator-associated pneumonia due to antibiotic-resistant gram-positive bacterial infection. Eur J Clin Microbiol Infect Dis 2005; 24:794–803.

Kreissler-Haag D, Schilling MK, Maurer CA. [Surgery of complicated gastroduodenal ulcers: outcome at the millennium]. Zentralbl Chir 2002; 127:1078–82.

Krobot K, Yin D, Zhang Q et al. Effect of inappropriate initial empiric antibiotic therapy on outcome of patients with community-acquired intra-abdominal infections requiring surgery. Eur J Clin Microbiol Infect Dis 2004; 23:682–7.

Kujath P, Schwandner O, Bruch HP. Morbidity and mortality of perforated peptic gastroduodenal ulcer following emergency surgery. Langenbecks Arch Surg 2002; 387:298–302.

Lamme B, Mahler CW, van Ruler O et al. Clinical predictors of ongoing infection in secondary peritonitis: systematic review. World J Surg 2006; 30:2170–81.

Lankisch PG, Mahlke R, Lübbers H. [Certified medical education: the acute abdomen from a medical point of view]. Dtsch Arztebl 2006; 103: A2179–88.

Lippert H, Koch A, Marusch F et al. [Open vs. laparoscopic appendectomy.] Chirurg 2002; 73:791–8.

Loo VG, Poirier L, Miller MA et al. A predominantly clonal multi-institutional outbreak of clostridium difficile–associated diarrhea with high morbidity and mortality. N Engl J Med 2005; 353:2442–9.

Lunevicius R, Morkevicius M. Risk factors influencing the early outcome results after laparoscopic repair of perforated duodenal ulcer and their predictive value. Langenbecks Arch Surg 2005; 390:413–20.

McDonald LC, Killgore GE, Thompson A et al. An epidemic, toxin gene–variant strain of clostridium difficile. N Engl J Med 2005; 353:2433–41.

MacFie J, Reddy BS, Gatt M et al. Bacterial translocation studied in 927 patients over 13 years. Br J Surg 2006; 93:87–93.

Manger T, Fahlke J, Pross M et al. [Laparoscopic cholecystectomy. A recommendable indication in acute cholecystitis?] Zentralbl Chir 1999; 124:1121–9.

Maroske D, Stroh M, Roher HD. [Early operation for acute gallbladder as a therapeutic principle.] Dtsch Med Wochenschr 1985; 110:1108–14.

Marshall JC. Intra-abdominal infections. Microbes Infect 2004; 6:1015–25.

Mazuski JE, Solomkin JS. Intra-abdominal infections. Surg Clin North Am 2009; 89:421–37.

Mazuski JE, Sawyer RG, Nathens AB et al. Therapeutic Agents Committee of the Surgical Infections Society. The Surgical Infection Society guidelines on antimicrobial therapy for intra-abdominal infections: evidence for the recommendations. Surg Infect (Larchmt) 2002; 3:175–233.

Montravers P, Gauzit R, Muller C et al. Emergence of antibiotic-resistant bacteria in cases of peritonitis after intraabdominal surgery affects the efficacy of empirical antimicrobial therapy. Clin Infect Dis 1996; 23:486–94.

Moyenuddin M, Williamson JC, Ohl CA. Clostridium difficile-associated diarrhea: current strategies for diagnosis and therapy. Curr Gastroenterol Rep 2002; 4:279-86 4:279–86.

Ohmann C, Wittman DH, Wacha H. Prospective evaluation of prognostic scoring systems in peritonitis: peritonitis study group. Eur J Surg 1993; 159:267–74.

Ohmann C, Yang Q, Hau T et al. Prognostic modeling in peritonitis: peritonitis study group of the surgical infection society europe. Eur J Surg 1997; 163:53–60.

Panhofer P, Izay B, Riedl M et al. Age, microbiology and prognostic scores help to differentiate between secondary and tertiary peritonitis. Langenbecks Arch Surg 2009; 394:265–71.

Paulson EK, Kalady MF, Pappas TN. Suspected appendicitis. N Engl J Med 2003; 348:236–42.

Privitera G, Scarpellini P, Prtisi G et al. Prospective study of Clostridium difficile intestinal colonization and disease following single-dose antibiotic prophylaxis in surgery. Antimicrob Agents Chemother 1991; 35:208–10.

Ranson J. Conservative surgical treatment of acute pancreatitis. World J Surg 1981; 5:351–9.

Ranson JH. Acute pancreatitis. Curr Probl Surg 1979; 16:1–84.

Richter S, Lindermann W, Kollmar O et al. One-stage sigmoid colon resection for perforated sigmoid diverticulitis (Hinchey stages III and IV). World J Surg 2006; 30:1027–32.

Robert JH, Frossard JL, Mermillod B et al. Early prediction of acute pancreatitis: prospective study comparing computed tomography scans, ranson, glascow, acute physiology and chronic health evaluation II scores, and various serum markers. World J Surg 2002; 26:612–9.

Rodriguez-Sanjuan JC, Fernandez-Santiago R, Garcia RA et al. Perforated peptic ulcer treated by simple closure and Helicobacter pylori eradication. World J Surg 2005; 29:849–52.

Röhrborn A, Wacha H, Schöffel U et al. Coverage of enterococci in community acquired secondary peritonitis: results of a randomized trial. Surg Infect (Larchmt) 2000; 1:95–107.

Sánchez-Navarro MD, Coloma Milano C, Zarzuelo Castañeda A et al. Pharmacokinetics of ciprofloxacin as a tool to optimise dosage schedules in community patients. Clin Pharmacokinet 2002; 41:1213–20.

Sawyer RG, Barkun JS, Smith R et al. Recognition and management of intra-abdominal infection. In: ACS Surgery: principles and practice. Edited by DW Wilmore. New York: WebMD, 2004; 1–29.

Schein M, Assalia A, Bachus H. Minimal antibiotic therapy after emergency abdominal surgery: a prospective study. Br J Surg 1994; 81:989–91.

Schroeder MS. Clostridium difficile-associated diarrhea. Am Fam Physician 2005; 71:921–8.

Schwarz M, Poch B, Isenmann R et al. Effect of early and late antibiotic treatment in experimental acute pancreatitis in rats. Langenbecks Arch Surg 2007; 392:365–70.

Sharma VK, Howden CW. Prophylactic antibiotic administration reduces sepsis and mortality in acute necrotizing pancreatitis: a meta-analysis. Pancreas 2001; 22:28–31.

Solomkin J, Teppler H, Graham DR et al. Treatment of polymicrobial infections: post hoc analysis of three trials comparing ertapenem and piperacillin-tazobactam. J Antimicrob Chemother (Suppl) 2004; 53:ii51–7.

Solomkin JS, Dellinger EP, Bohnen JM et al. The role of oral antimicrobials for the management of intra-abdominal infections. New Horiz (Suppl)1998; 6:S46–52.

Solomkin JS, Reinhart HH, Dellinger EP et al. Results of a randomized trial comparing sequential intravenous/oral treatment with ciprofloxacin plus metronidazole to imipenem/cilastatin for intra-abdominal infections. The intra-abdominal infection study group. Ann Surg 1996; 223:303–315.

Solomkin JS, Yellin AE, Rotstein OD et al. Ertapenem versus piperacillin/tazobactam in the treatment of complicated intraabdominal infections: results of a double-blind, randomized comparative phase III trial. Ann Surg 2003; 237:235–45.

Solomkin JS, Dellinger EP, Christou NV et al. Results of a multicenter trial comparing imipenem/ cilastatin to tobramycin/clindamycin for intra-abdominal infections. Ann Surg 1990; 212:581–91.

Song F, Glenny AM. Antimicrobial prophylaxis in colorectal surgery: a systematic review of randomized controlled trials. Br J Surg 1998; 85: 1232–41.

Søreide K, Kørner H, Søreide JA. Type II error in a randomized controlled trial of appendectomy vs. antibiotic treatment of acute appendicitis. World J Surg 2007; 31:871–2.

Sotto A, Lefrant JY, Fabbro-Peray P et al. Evaluation of antimicrobial therapy management of 120 consecutive patients with secondary peritonitis. J Antimicrob Chemother 2002; 50:569–76.

Steinberg W. Gastroenterology and hepatology: pancreas. Edited by M Feldman, PP Toskes. Philadelphia: Current Medicine LLC: 1998.

Stone HH, Bourneuf AA, Stinson LD. Reliability of criteria for predicting persistent or recurrent sepsis. Arch Surg 1985; 120:17–20.

Styrud J, Eriksson S, Nilsson I et al. Appendectomy versus antibiotic treatment in acute appendicitis. A prospective multicenter randomized controlled trial. World J Surg 2006; 30:1033–7.

Surgical Infection Society and the Infectious Diseases Society of America. Solomin JS, Mazuski JE, Bradley JS et al. Diagnosis and Management of Complicated Intra-abdominal Infection in Adults and Children: Guidelines by the Surgical Infection Society and the Infectious Diseases Society of America. Clin Infect Dis 2010; 50:133–64.

Teppler H, McCarroll K, Gesser RM et al. Surgical infections with enterococcus: outcome in patients treated with ertapenem versus piperacillin-tazobactam. Surg Infect (Larchmt) 2002; 3:337–49.

Thomas DR. Conservative management of the appendix mass. Surgery 1973; 73:677–80.

Urbach DR, Marshall JC. Pancreatic abscess and infected pancreatic necrosis. Curr Opin Surg Infect 1996; 4:57–66.

Van Lent AU, Bartelsman JF, Tytgat GN et al. Duration of antibiotic therapy for cholangitis after successful endoscopic drainage of the biliary tract. Gastrointest Endosc 2002; 55:518–22.

Wacha H, Schäffer V, Schöffer U et al. [Peritonitis and other intra-abdominal infections]. In: Die Infektiologie. Edited by D Adam, HW Doerr, H Link, H Lode. Berlin: Springer, 2004; 333–52.

Wacha H, Hau T, Dittmer R et al. Risk factors associated with intra-abdominal infections: a prospective multicenter study. Langenbecks Arch Surg 1999; 384:24–32.

Wacha H, Helm EB. Efficacy of antibiotics in bacteriobilia. J Antimicrob Chemother (Suppl) 1982; 9:131–7.

Wacha H, Interwies E. Peritonitis -Grundsätzliches zur Therapie. Berlin: Springer-Verlag GmbH, 1987.

Wacha H, Rieber W, Schumann J et al. [Pathogen elimination after surgical interventions on common bile duct.] Langenbecks Arch Chirg 1979; 350:59–63.

Wacha H, Warren B, Bassaris H et al. The Intra-abdominal Infections Study Group. Comparison of sequential intravenous/oral ciprofloxacin plus metronidazole with intravenous ceftriaxone plus metronidazole for treatment of complicated intra-abdominal infections. Surg Infect (Larchmt) 2006; 7:341–54.

Wilcox C. Gastroenterology and hepatology: stomach and duodenum. Edited by M Feldman, Philadelphia: Current Medicine LLC, 1996.

Zar FA, Bakkanagari SR, Moorthi K et al. A Comparison of vancomycin and metronidazole for the treatment of clostridium difficile–associated diarrhea, stratified by disease severity. Clin Infect Dis 2007; 45:302– 7.

Zeitoun G, Laurent A, Rouffet et al. Multicentre, randomized clinical trial of primary versus secondary sigmoid resection in generalized peritonitis complicating sigmoid diverticulitis. Br J Surg 2000; 87:1366–74.